A Note to the Teacher

Chapter Tests

Chapter Tests consist of matching, multiple choice, short answer, and essay items that assess students' mastery of the objectives for each chapter. A complete answer key is provided in the back of this book.

Alternative Assessments

The Alternative Assessments use alternative methods, such as hands-on learning and personal experience, to assess whether students have mastered certain chapter concepts. These worksheets are also designed to test the students' abilities to apply knowledge and life-management skills. The Alternative Assessment can be used in conjunction with other assessment methods to develop a portfolio assessment plan.

Many of the questions and assignments in the Alternative Assessment worksheets ask for students' opinions or personal experiences and do not have correct answers. In these cases, the answer key in the back of this book may provide sample answers or suggest ways to evaluate student effort. After the assessment, you may wish to discuss with each student his or her strengths and weaknesses.

Table of Contents

Alternative Assessments

NAME ________________ CLASS ______ DATE ______

Health and Wellness: A Quality of Life
Chapter Test

Part I

Match the definitions on the right with the terms on the left.

_____ **1.** communicable disease

_____ **2.** emotional health

_____ **3.** mental health

_____ **4.** physical fitness

_____ **5.** physical health

_____ **6.** self-esteem

_____ **7.** social health

_____ **8.** social support

_____ **9.** spiritual health

_____ **10.** wellness

a. aspects of health related to the body

b. involves interacting well with people and having satisfying relationships

c. feeling good about oneself

d. an illness passed from person to person by an organism

e. having a sense of self-worth and the ability to tolerate differences

f. ability to control and appropriately express feelings

g. ability to find peace with yourself and with those around you

h. achieved by looking at your total health from a positive perspective

i. using others to share life experiences and situations

j. a state in which your body can meet the daily demands of living

Part II

Read each situation below. Determine the health of each person. Indicate where each person would fall on the health-illness continuum by writing the number of the statement in the appropriate blank space below the continuum.

Health-Illness Continuum

Death — Illness — Average health — Emotional growth — Optimal health or wellness

_____ _____ _____ _____ _____

11. Sonya smokes a pack of cigarettes a day. She coughs every morning and has had five colds this past winter.

12. Daryl's girlfriend just broke up with him. This was Daryl's first relationship, and he feels sad and hurt. Daryl has decided that he will get over his sadness by doing something he enjoys and by keeping in mind that he will find someone else.

13. Jennifer exercises and eats a well-balanced diet. She maintains friendships and is able to deal with and meet the demands of everyday life.

14. Jason drove while he was drunk and was involved in a serious car accident. He is now in a coma and hooked up to several machines.

15. Whitney is a teenager and sometimes feels overwhelmed and confused by the physical and emotional changes her body is going through. However, when she feels this way she talks with people she can trust for support. Whitney is a few pounds above her ideal weight. She hopes to lose the weight by starting an exercise program and by eating a better diet.

Part III ·

Write the letter of the correct answer in the blank.

_____ **16.** Manuel is a well-adjusted person. He maintains friendships, controls stress, deals with every-day problems, exercises, and eats a balanced diet. Manuel feels good about himself and is able to make decisions that maximize his health. Manuel has

    a. physical health   c. good self-esteem
    b. average health   d. wellness

_____ **17.** Being physically fit enables a person to

    a. prevent certain diseases, such as heart disease
    b. feel good about himself or herself
    c. have strength and endurance
    d. all of the above

_____ **18.** In order to have optimal health, you do not need

    a. physical health   c. positive self-esteem
    b. good relationships   d. psychological counseling

_____ **19.** The leading cause of death among teenagers when your great-grandparents were your age was

    a. homicide   c. diseases
    b. car accidents   d. suicide

_____ **20.** The leading cause of death among teenagers today is

    a. homicide   c. diseases
    b. car accidents   d. suicide

_____ **21.** The disease that causes the most deaths among adult Americans is

    a. heart disease   c. pneumonia and influenza
    b. cancer   d. lung disease

_____ **22.** A health issue teenagers face today is

    a. depression   c. sexually transmitted diseases
    b. suicide   d. all of the above

_____ **23.** Many of the leading causes of death among teenagers and adults can be prevented through

    a. changes in the environment
    b. new and better medical treatment
    c. lifestyle changes
    d. better diets

Part IV . . . .

Write the answers to the questions in the spaces provided.

24. Your friend Rob smokes cigarettes, occasionally uses marijuana, and drinks alcohol at parties. He also engages in sexual intercourse without protection. He says none of these behaviors are harming him because he feels fine. What could you tell him?

25. What four guidelines can you follow now to positively affect your future quality of health?

Chapter 2

Making Responsible Decisions
Chapter Test

Part I ....

Match the definitions on the left with the terms on the right.

_____ **1.** The number of years a person can reasonably expect to live

_____ **2.** The degree to which a person lives life to its fullest capacity with enjoyment and reward

_____ **3.** The killing of one person by another

_____ **4.** The act of intentionally killing oneself

_____ **5.** A person's strong beliefs and ideals

_____ **6.** A series of steps that help a person make a responsible decision

a. decision-making model

b. homicide

c. life expectancy

d. quality of life

e. suicide

f. values

Part II ....

Write the letter of the correct answer on the line provided.

_____ **7.** The leading cause of death among people aged 15 to 24 is
- a. suicide
- b. homicide
- c. unintentional injury
- d. drug overdose

_____ **8.** A major cause of death among people aged 15 to 24 is
- a. cancer
- b. suicide
- c. alcoholism
- d. heart disease

_____ **9.** Which of the following behaviors can put a person at risk of unintentional injury?
- a. drinking alcohol
- b. using drugs
- c. not using seat belts
- d. all of the above

_____ **10.** The leading cause of death among people aged 55 to 64 is
- a. heart disease
- b. cancer
- c. stroke
- d. unintentional injury

_____ **11.** Which of the following behaviors can decrease a person's quality of life?
- a. smoking
- b. exercising
- c. low-fat diet
- d. all of the above

_____ **12.** Which of the following factors contributes most to death rates in the United States?
- a. inadequate health care
- b. heredity
- c. unhealthful lifestyles
- d. environment

_____ **13.** When listing options, you should list
     a. those that first come to mind
     b. all options given to you by other people
     c. options that come to you after giving more thought to the problem
     d. all of the above

_____ **14.** As you consider your options when making a decision, you do *not* need to be governed by
     a. your values   c. what you have done in the past
     b. the consequences of your behavior   d. the benefits of your behavior

_____ **15.** A good decision
     a. always works out well   c. tries to control other people's behaviors
     b. is one that is made responsibly   d. a and b

_____ **16.** Following the decision-making steps enables you to
     a. act responsibly
     b. make responsible decisions quickly, if you need to
     c. consider your values first
     d. all of the above

Part III ·

**Listed below are some behaviors. Write S on the line in front of the behaviors
that have short-term consequences. Write L on the line in front of the behaviors
that have long-term consequences. Some behaviors may have both short-term
and long-term consequences.**

_____ **17.** Drinking alcohol

_____ **18.** Using drugs

_____ **19.** Smoking

_____ **20.** Wearing a bicycle helmet

_____ **21.** Eating a poor diet

_____ **22.** Getting little exercise

Part IV ·

Answer the questions using complete sentences.

**You meet Seth at a party. After talking for a while, you feel that you would like
to become friends with him. He then pulls out a pack of cigarettes. As he lights
one, Seth asks if you would like a cigarette also.**

23. What are your options?

____

____

____

24. What are the benefits and negative consequences of these options?

25. What are your values concerning smoking?

26. What is your decision?

27. How would you carry out your decision?

Physical Fitness

Chapter Test

Part I

Match the definitions on the right with the terms on the left.

_____ **1.** aerobic exercise

_____ **2.** anaerobic exercise

_____ **3.** body composition

_____ **4.** cholesterol

_____ **5.** high blood pressure

_____ **6.** insomnia

_____ **7.** physical fitness

_____ **8.** REM

_____ **9.** steroid

_____ **10.** endorphins

_____ **11.** muscular strength

_____ **12.** aerobic fitness

a. the ability to endure at least 10 minutes of moderate activity

b. a condition in which the blood pushes harder than normal against the inside of the blood vessels

c. the ability to perform daily tasks vigorously, the ability to perform physical activities and exercise, and the capacity to avoid diseases related to a lack of activity

d. physical activity that increases the supply of oxygen to the body and that can be continued for a period of time without resting

e. an artificially made substance that can temporarily increase muscle size

f. the dreaming part of the sleep cycle in which the eyes move back and forth rapidly under the eyelids

g. substances produced inside the brain that have pleasurable effects

h. physical activity that increases speed and muscular strength

i. the division of the total body weight into fat weight and muscle weight

j. temporary or continuing loss of sleep

k. a waxy, fatty substance that can block the arteries and cause heart disease

l. the muscles' ability to push against a very heavy force over a short period of time

Part II

Write the letter of the correct answer in the blank.

_____ **13.** Exercise is important because exercise can help you
   a. lose weight
   b. cope better with stress
   c. increase your energy level
   d. all of the above

_____ **14.** A physical benefit of exercise is
   a. increase in muscle size
   b. increase in heart strength
   c. increase in bone strength
   d. all of the above

_______ **15.** Exercise is beneficial to the heart because exercise
    a. raises blood cholesterol
    b. increases heart strength
    c. raises blood pressure
    d. all of the above

_______ **16.** A person who is physically fit
    a. has a high level of endorphins
    b. experiences mood swings
    c. has muscular strength and endurance
    d. needs increased steroids

_______ **17.** To test for aerobic fitness, you can
    a. do sit-ups   c. do pull-ups
    b. walk one mile quickly   d. all of the above

_______ **18.** If you are physically fit, during the body composition test you should be able to pinch no more than
    a. three inches from your abdomen
    b. two inches from your thigh
    c. one inch on your upper arm
    d. all of the above

_______ **19.** Carlos walked one mile and had a heart rate of 60 beats per minute. He could do 40 sit-ups in one minute. But when Carlos sat with his feet straight out in front of him and bent at his waist to touch his feet, he found he could not do so. Carlos needs to improve his
    a. flexibility   c. muscle strength
    b. body composition   d. aerobic fitness

_______ **20.** An example of aerobic exercise is
    a walking   c. swimming
    b. cycling   d. all of the above

_______ **21.** An example of anaerobic exercise is
    a. baseball   c. weight lifting
    b. bowling   d. all of the above

_______ **22.** A rule to follow when exercising is
    a. always ignore pain
    b. always dress for the weather
    c. wear a rubberized suit when exercising to lose weight
    d. plan to work out strenuously only one day a week

_______ **23.** Knowing your target heart rate can help you determine if you are exercising at the proper intensity. Your target heart rate should be about how many beats per minute?
    a. 250   c. 160
    b. 185   d. 110

Part III ●

Answer the question in the space provided.

24. A friend of yours is thinking of taking steroids to increase muscle size. What would you advise your friend to do? Why?

Chapter 4

Nutrition Principles

Chapter Test

Part I

Match the definitions on the right with the terms on the left.

_____ **1.** appetite

_____ **2.** cholesterol

_____ **3.** hunger

_____ **4.** nutrient

_____ **5.** nutrition

a. the study of the way in which substances affect one's health

b. the body's physical response to the need for food

c. the desire to eat based on the pleasure you get from eating certain foods

d. a substance generally obtained from food that is necessary for the carrying out of body functions

e. a fatlike substance that is part of cell membranes

Part II

Use the terms from the following list to complete each sentence below. A term may be used only once. Some terms will not be used at all.

appetite	aroma	culture	emotions
health	hunger	religion	weather

6. Elizabeth and Miriam are shopping at the mall. Miriam is hungry. Elizabeth isn't hungry but agrees to get some food. Miriam orders stir-fried rice. Elizabeth orders some too.

Elizabeth's choice to order food is influenced by _______________________.

7. Jason has the flu and is experiencing nausea. His sister asks him if he would like some chicken noodle soup. Jason says, "No, thanks." His decision is influenced by

_______________________.

8. Manuel is getting ready for school. His mother asks him if he would like some waffles and turkey sausage for breakfast. He says, "Yes, that sounds great. I didn't eat much for dinner

last night." Manuel's decision is influenced by _______________________.

9. Isabel grew up in the southern United States. When she was 12, she moved to the West Coast. After eating dinner in a restaurant, she noticed they were serving homemade pecan pie made with Georgia pecans. Isabel felt she just had to order a piece of the pie. Her

decision was influenced by _______________________.

10. Mike found out he did not make the basketball team. That evening, Mike's friends invited him out for pizza. Mike went with his friends but did not eat very much of the pizza. Mike's

decision not to eat much was influenced by _______________________.

Part III

Write the letter of the correct answer in the blank.

_______ **11.** A short-term consequence of poor nutrition is
    a. fatigue
    b. illness
    c. obesity
    d. tooth decay

_______ **12.** A long-term consequence of poor nutrition is
    a. depression
    b. fatigue
    c. illness
    d. loss of concentration

_______ **13.** The main food source for energy comes from
    a. carbohydrates
    b. proteins
    c. fats
    d. minerals

_______ **14.** The substance that is necessary for the production of certain hormones and that helps store and transport vitamins is
    a. carbohydrates
    b. water
    c. proteins
    d. fats

_______ **15.** The substance that is essential for body growth and repair is
    a. vitamins
    b. fats
    c. proteins
    d. carbohydrates

_______ **16.** A deficiency of calcium can lead to
    a. rickets
    b. osteoporosis
    c. scurvy
    d. anemia

_______ **17.** For a healthful diet, nutrients need to be consumed in different amounts. For example, carbohydrates should
    a. be limited to 300 milligrams a day
    b. make up about 30 percent of your daily caloric intake
    c. be limited to 3000 milligrams a day
    d. make up about 50 percent of your daily caloric intake

_______ **18.** A substance that carries fats from the digestive system to body cells and is associated with an increased risk of coronary artery disease is
    a. fats from fruits, nuts, and vegetables
    b. unsaturated fats
    c. low-density lipoproteins
    d. high-density lipoproteins

_______ **19.** The Reference Daily Intakes (RDI)
    a. replaced the formerly used RDAs
    b. are the accepted nutrition standard for Americans
    c. are useful in planning meals
    d. all of the above

_______ **20.** Food-borne illnesses usually affect

    a. the extremities
    b. the stomach and the intestines
    c. the liver and the kidneys
    d. the circulatory system

_______ **21.** Foods that can be affected by bacteria

    a. should be bought at the end of a shopping trip
    b. include fish and poultry
    c. include eggs, even though they have a shell
    d. all of the above

_______ **22.** Bread is rich in complex carbohydrates and is a low-fat source of fiber, minerals, and vitamins. Usually, the more fiber in the bread, the more nutrients. Look at the following labels of four loaves of bread:

	calories	sodium	fiber
loaf 1:	60	100 mg	1 g
loaf 2:	70	160 mg	2 g
loaf 3:	40	105 mg	2 g
loaf 4:	80	5 mg	3 g

Which loaf of bread is the most nutritious choice?
    a. loaf 1   c. loaf 3
    b. loaf 2   d. loaf 4

_______ **23.** Which of the following meals is the most nutritious?

    a. Pasta with creamed alfredo sauce, toasted garlic bread, tossed salad
    b. Broiled fish, steamed carrots, brown and wild rice
    c. Fried eggs, bacon, buttered toast and jelly
    d. Beef tacos with sour cream and cheddar cheese, refried beans, rice

_______ **24.** Skim milk is a good choice for protein, vitamin D, and calcium. Which group would have the greatest need for including milk in their diet?

    a. Adults   c. Teenagers
    b. Vegetarians   d. Athletes

Part IV ·

25. Lydia usually skips breakfast and eats a bag of potato chips and a milkshake for lunch. Her favorite foods for dinner are hamburgers, hot dogs, and pizza. What is wrong with Lydia's diet? How can she change her diet to better meet her nutritional needs?

____

____

____

____

____

Chapter 5

Weight Management and Eating Disorders

Chapter Test

Part I

Match the terms on the left with the definitions on the right.

_____ **1.** basal metabolic rate

_____ **2.** binge

_____ **3.** constipation

_____ **4.** diarrhea

_____ **5.** lean mass

_____ **6.** metabolism

_____ **7.** obese

_____ **8.** overweight

_____ **9.** pica

a. how the body breaks down food so it can be used for energy and other purposes

b. the rate at which the body uses energy when it is at rest

c. weighing 10 percent more than one's recommended weight

d. weighing 20 percent more than one's recommended weight

e. total body weight minus weight due to fat

f. involves eating substances not normally considered to be food

g. involves eating large amounts of food over a short time

h. frequent bowel movements that are loose and watery

i. difficult or infrequent bowel movements

Part II

Write the letter of the correct answer in the blank.

_____ **10.** Hershel is very active. He exercises every day. To determine what his caloric intake should be, Hershel needs to

    a. know his body composition
    b. calculate his percentage of body fat
    c. determine his energy balance
    d. know his activity level

_____ **11.** Ideal body weight should be based on

    a. height and weight charts
    b. body composition
    c. size of body frame
    d. lean mass

_____ **12.** Peter is obese. He wants to lose 50 pounds. Which of the following is a safe and reasonable way to reach this goal?

    a. Start a diet plan he saw advertised in a magazine
    b. Make an appointment with his doctor to discuss a weight-loss plan
    c. Cut all fatty foods from his diet
    d. Cut all snacks from his diet and drink only water or diet drinks

_____ 13. Rosalind wants to gain some weight. A good way for her to do this is to
 a. eat foods high in fat
 b. snack often and close to meals
 c. begin exercising or increase her activity level
 d. begin taking a supplement that guarantees weight gain

_____ 14. Your sister is pregnant. Before the pregnancy, she was overweight. Your sister wants to try to control her weight now and gain only 15 pounds, despite her doctor's advice. Your sister may be at risk for
 a. delivering a low-weight baby who could have health problems
 b. developing anorexia nervosa or bulimia
 c. developing pica
 d. developing digestive disorders

_____ 15. Digestive problems can be caused by
 a. overeating   c. food intolerance
 b. a food allergy   d. all of the above

_____ 16. A healthful and efficient way to treat a single case of constipation is to
 a. take a laxative
 b. consult with your doctor
 c. add more high-fiber food to your diet
 d. all of the above

_____ 17. James notices that when he eats cucumbers he experiences gas and bloating along with heartburn, or indigestion. James is experiencing
 a. food allergy   c. food intolerance
 b. anaphylactic shock   d. dehydration

_____ 18. Susan has an allergic reaction whenever she eats foods that have been treated with sulfites. An allergic symptom Susan may experience is
 a. cramping   c. constipation
 b. tightening in the throat   d. imbalance in electrolytes

Part III

Write A on the line next to the statement that represents a characteristic of anorexia nervosa. Write B on the line next to the statement that represents a characteristic of bulimia. Some statements may be characteristic of both disorders.

_____ 19. Constant dieting that is carried to an extreme

_____ 20. Frequent use of laxatives

_____ 21. State of starvation

_____ 22. Binge-purge cycle

_____ 23. Refusing to eat

_____ 24. Low self-esteem

Part IV . . . .

Answer the question in the space provided.

25. You are creating a healthful weight-loss diet and a healthful weight-gain diet. Would you include fast food in either of your diets? If so, in which diet(s)? Explain why you would or would not include fast food in your diet plans.

Chapter 6

Personal Care and Appearance

Chapter Test

Part I

Match the definitions on the right with the terms on the left.

______ **1.** calculus

______ **2.** dermis

______ **3.** enamel

______ **4.** epidermis

______ **5.** melanin

______ **6.** plaque

a. the very thin outer layer of the skin

b. the second layer of skin; contains the most important structures of the skin

c. the substance covering the crown of the tooth

d. a film of food particles, saliva, and bacteria on the teeth

e. hardened plaque

f. the substance that protects the skin from the sun's rays; also produces freckles

Part II

Write the letter of the correct answer in the blank.

______ **7.** The main function of the subcutaneous layer of skin is to
   a. protect the body from germs
   b. insulate the body from temperature changes
   c. produce melanin
   d. transmit sensations, such as pain

______ **8.** Pimples are a form of skin blemish. Pimples
   a. form when a clogged pore becomes infected
   b. form when oil and dead skin cells clog a pore and are exposed to air
   c. can be totally prevented
   d. a and c

______ **9.** A person can reduce his or her chance of developing acne by
   a. using oil-based makeup
   b. washing the face several times a day
   c. exposing the face to sunlight
   d. squeezing pimples that appear

______ **10.** A condition that is characterized by skin that flakes off the scalp is
   a. ringworm   c. dandruff
   b. balding   d. head lice

______ **11.** Ringworm is a skin condition that is caused by a
   a. bacterial infection   c. fungus
   b. parasitic worm   d. none of the above

_______ **12.** To keep your hair healthy and to help improve your appearance, you can
     a. wash your hair regularly
     b. avoid sharing combs, brushes, or towels
     c. brush your hair daily
     d. all of the above

_______ **13.** To keep your nails healthy, you can
     a. file the nails in a back-and-forth motion
     b. cut fingernails so they are slightly rounded
     c. soak your nails for 20 minutes once a week in a soap-and-water solution
     d. all of the above

_______ **14.** The major cause of cavities is
     a. calculus   c. poor alignment of teeth
     b. plaque buildup   d. flossing every other day

_______ **15.** Poor alignment of teeth can be corrected through
     a. improvement in diet
     b. removal of tartar from the teeth
     c. use of braces
     d. brushing twice a day

_______ **16.** To maintain healthy teeth and gums, you should
     a. brush twice a day and floss once a day
     b. clean off calculus daily
     c. avoid mouthwashes
     d. see your dentist when you have a cavity

_______ **17.** To find a dentist to care for your oral health, you could
     a. use the Yellow Pages
     b. ask your friends who their dentists are and how well they like their dentists
     c. call a dentist/physician referral service
     d. all of the above

Part III

Match the skin conditions on the left with the definitions on the right.

_______ **18.** acne

_______ **19.** wart

_______ **20.** athlete's foot

_______ **21.** impetigo

_______ **22.** sunburn

_______ **23.** mole

a. redness of the skin caused by excessive exposure to ultraviolet light

b. condition caused when pores become clogged with oil

c. fungal infection that causes redness and itching

d. small growth caused by a virus

e. a bacterial infection that causes sores with crusts on the skin

f. a small, round, dark area on the skin

Part IV ·

Answer the question in the space provided.

24. It is a hot, sunny summer day. You ask your friend, Anita, to go to a 12:30 P.M. movie. Anita tells you she won't be able to go because she plans to sunbathe in her backyard from 11:00 A.M. to 2:00 P.M. She says she wants to get a deep tan, so she will be applying baby oil to her skin. Is Anita making a healthful decision? Why or why not?

____

____

____

____

____

____

25. List the precautions you should take if you suspect that you have come into contact with poison ivy, poison sumac, or poison oak.

____

____

____

____

____

____

____

Chapter 7

Mental and Emotional Health
Chapter Test

Part I ....
Match the definitions on the right with the correct terms on the left.

_____ **1.** behavior modification

_____ **2.** defense mechanisms

_____ **3.** emotions

_____ **4.** mental health

_____ **5.** dissociative disorder

_____ **6.** psychoanalysis

_____ **7.** somatoform disorder

_____ **8.** self-concept

_____ **9.** self-esteem

_____ **10.** self-ideal

a. meeting the demands of life

b. a realistic image to strive for

c. feelings in response to an activity or an experience

d. techniques used to protect oneself from being hurt

e. self-image

f. feeling good about yourself and the things you do

g. a functional disorder in which people separate themselves from their real personality

h. techniques used to reward desirable behavior

i. a functional disorder in which the person has physical symptoms caused by emotional problems

j. techniques used to examine unresolved conflicts from the past

Part II ....
Write the letter of the correct answer in the blank.

_____ **11.** Which of the following is *not* a characteristic of a mentally healthy person?
   a. Feels good about himself or herself
   b. Is optimistic
   c. Finds ways to keep in contact with friends and make new friends
   d. Always avoids difficult or unpleasant situations

_____ **12.** Happiness is an emotion that can be achieved. To become a happy person, one
   a. must experience romantic love
   b. needs to learn to control anger by ignoring those feelings
   c. should focus on positive things in his or her life
   d. should use defense mechanisms whenever possible

_____ **13.** Joseph just had an argument with his girlfriend. He was angry. However, he has learned to express his anger in a positive way. When Joseph got home, he
   a. yelled at his younger sister and her friends because they were laughing too loud and he could not hear the television
   b. changed into some old, comfortable clothes and rode his bicycle
   c. went to his room and punched the wall several times with his fists
   d. decided it might be best to break up with his girlfriend because it is her attitude that always causes their arguments

_____ **14.** Mary failed her history test. When her parents asked why that happened, Mary told them it was the teacher's fault. The teacher asked too many questions on subjects that were not covered in lecture. What defense mechanism is Mary using to cope with her failing grade?

    a. Denial   c. Projection
    b. Displacement   d. Rationalization

_____ **15.** Angelina has just won first place in an ice-skating competition. She feels good about her success on the ice. She likes to share her good feelings and enjoyment of ice skating by volunteering some time every week to teach handicapped children how to skate. According to Maslow's hierarchy of needs, Angelina is at the level known as

    a. safety-security   c. self-esteem
    b. love and affection   d. self-actualization

_____ **16.** Electra has taken on too many responsibilities. She told you that lately she hasn't been able to sleep, eat, concentrate, or make decisions. Who could you talk to in order to get help for Electra?

    a. A druggist
    b. A neurologist
    c. A substance-abuse counselor
    d. A school nurse

_____ **17.** Samuel plays aggressively with other children. Whenever he plays rough, his mother makes him sit in a chair for five minutes. Whenever he plays nicely, his mother gives him a sticker. When Samuel gets 10 stickers he trades them in for a fruit-juice bar. What is his mother using to deal with Samuel's aggression?

    a. Behavior therapy   c. Chemical therapy
    b. Psychoanalysis   d. Group therapy

Part III

Use the terms from the following list to correctly complete each sentence below. A term may be used only once. Some terms will not be used.

antisocial personality disorder	paranoid personality disorder
hypochondriasis	passive-aggressive personality disorder
manic-depressive disorder	phobia
multiple personality disorder	schizophrenia
organic disorder	

18. Jason is terrified of spiders. Whenever he sees one, he must get away as quickly as possible. Jason

has a(n) _______________________________.

19. Brenda was sexually abused as a child. As an adult, her personality can change dramatically, as if she becomes a different person. Sometimes she is shy and timid; at other times she is outspoken and

aggressive. Brenda may have _______________________________.

20. Sometimes Stephanie is extremely excited, happy, and full of energy. At other times, she seems

dangerously sad and depressed. Stephanie could have _______________________________.

21. Thomas thinks that everyone is against him. He trusts no one. Thomas may have

_______________________________.

22. Helen always seems to be complaining of some ache or pain, insisting that she is ill. She changes doctors frequently because none can find anything wrong with her. Helen may have

_______________________________________.

23. Michael was becoming very forgetful and was experiencing mood swings. After running several tests, his doctor found a small brain tumor. Michael has a(n) _______________________________________.

24. Billy prefers to do things by himself. He cares little for anyone else and doesn't respect the feelings of others. Billy may have _______________________________________.

Part IV . . . .
Answer the question in the space provided.

25. Sometimes you feel anxious just before a test and you worry whether or not you have studied hard enough. But you always get over these feelings once you begin the test and find out that you do know the answers to the test questions. Should you seek help? Explain.

____

____

____

____

____

Building Self-Esteem

Chapter Test

Part I . . . .

Match the terms on the left with the definitions on the right.

_____ **1.** body image

_____ **2.** integrity

_____ **3.** peer pressure

_____ **4.** positive self-talk

_____ **5.** self-disclosure

_____ **6.** self-esteem

_____ **7.** support group

a. pride in and acceptance of oneself

b. how a person sees his or her appearance, fitness, and health

c. a group of people who trust each other and are able to talk openly with each other

d. talking to oneself in a positive way about one's characteristics and abilities

e. telling another person meaningful information about oneself

f. the influence of a social group on an individual member of the group

g. firm belief and adherence to a code of moral values

Part II . . . .

Write the letter of the correct answer in the blank.

_____ **8.** When a person has a high self-esteem, he or she
   a. feels self-confident
   b. is able to give and receive love
   c. is able to make good decisions
   d. all of the above

_____ **9.** The development of self-esteem begins at
   a. birth   c. age 13
   b. age 3   d. age 16

_____ **10.** The development of self-esteem can be influenced by
   a. parents   c. the media
   b. peers   d. all of the above

_____ **11.** The media can affect one's self-esteem by only showing people
   a. who always look beautiful
   b. who are tall and thin
   c. having "perfect" bodies
   d. all of the above

______ **12.** Michael thinks that a "perfect" man should be tall, strong, muscular, and ruggedly handsome. Michael's idea of such a body image is most likely influenced by

a. magazine advertisements
b. television advertisements
c. popular movies
d. all of the above

______ **13.** Daniele is short and about 15 pounds above her ideal weight. She is always well-groomed and neatly dressed. Daniele is willing to try new activities because she is not afraid of failing. Which of the following is true of Daniele?

a. She has high self-esteem.
b. She has low self-esteem.
c. She has allowed the media to influence her self-esteem.
d. She has allowed negative comments about her height and weight to influence her self-esteem.

______ **14.** In evaluating self-esteem and body image it is important to remember that success comes

a. only to people who have ideal male or female body types
b. only to those who are wealthy
c. to people of all ethnicities and body types
d. all of the above

______ **15.** A person's self-esteem

a. cannot be changed
b. can be changed
c. is not important for being successful
d. does not influence his or her behavior

______ **16.** After evaluating his body image and self-esteem, Herschel decided he wanted to improve his physical image. To do so, Herschel might consider changing his

a. diet
b. exercise habits
c. grooming habits
d. all of the above

______ **17.** Which of the following is not an important step in raising your self-esteem?

a. deciding what to change
b. not judging yourself by unrealistic standards
c. comparing yourself to others
d. accepting yourself

______ **18.** Reginald has decided to accept himself instead of trying to be like others. By accepting himself, Reginald has

a. learned to see himself as a special and unique person
b. realistically assessed his strengths and weaknesses
c. stopped judging himself using media standards
d. all of the above

______ **19.** One way to raise your self-esteem is to

a. use positive self-talk
b. try to do something you can't do well
c. blame others for your feelings
d. criticize yourself for not meeting high standards

_____ **20.** Carla decided not to accept a glass of beer from Joe. Joe responded by saying, "Go ahead, be a wallflower," and walking away. Carla thought to herself, *I'm sorry Joe feels that way, but I don't need to drink to enjoy myself.* Which of the following is true of Carla?

    a. She has high self-esteem.
    b. She used positive self-talk.
    c. She resisted peer pressure.
    d. All of the above

_____ **21.** A support group can help you develop and maintain a positive self-esteem by

    a. pointing out all of your faults
    b. allowing you to talk openly and not exerting pressure on you
    c. sharing things you said with people outside the group
    d. all of the above

_____ **22.** Self-disclosure plays a central role in the development of positive self-esteem because it

    a. allows others to correct any distortions a person may have about himself or herself
    b. develops a person's self-reliance
    c. makes a person critical of other people
    d. all of the above

_____ **23.** Individuals with high self-esteem

    a. look out only for themselves
    b. manipulate or take advantage of others
    c. act with integrity
    d. all of the above

_____ **24.** You can raise your self-esteem by

    a. making a list of all your good qualities
    b. maintaining a positive attitude
    c. avoiding trying to change things you have no control over
    d. all of the above

Part III ·

Answer the question in the space provided.

25. Jalene sat on the bleachers watching the other students play a friendly game of basketball. One of the girls came over and asked Jalene to join them. Jalene said, "No thanks, I'll just watch." Then Jalene thought to herself, *Basketball is a hard game to play. I'm no good at basketball because I'm short. Everyone will think I look like a short clown. Besides, it's hard to make new friends.*

Name two things that Jalene is allowing to influence her self-esteem negatively. Suppose you were Jalene. What might you think about playing basketball if you had high self-esteem?

____

____

____

____

____

Managing Stress
Chapter Test

Part I ●

Match the terms on the left with the definitions on the right.

_______ **1.** selective awareness

_______ **2.** stress

_______ **3.** stressor

_______ **4.** stress intervention

_______ **5.** stress response

_______ **6.** support group

a. combination of a stressor and a stress response

b. any action that prevents a stressor from resulting in negative consequences

c. any new or potentially unpleasant situation

d. the body's reaction to a stressor

e. group of people who trust one another and are able to talk to one another about their problems

f. focusing on the aspects of a situation that help a person to feel better

Part II ●

Write the letter of the best answer in the blank.

_______ **7.** Physical signs of stress can include

    a. headaches   c. anger
    b. laughing   d. all of the above

_______ **8.** Emotional and mental signs of stress can include

    a. mood swings   c. confusion
    b. nightmares   d. all of the above

_______ **9.** Jack is trying out for the baseball team. He is next at bat. His heart is racing and his palms are beginning to sweat. Jack is experiencing a

    a. loss of self-confidence   c. stressor
    b. stress response   d. all of the above

_______ **10.** Stressors can involve

    a. self-esteem   c. daily routines
    b. positive situations   d. all of the above

_______ **11.** Prolonged stress can

    a. make a person more susceptible to colds and flu
    b. cause tension headaches
    c. contribute to coronary heart disease
    d. all of the above

_______ **12.** The stress response can
      a. at times be helpful
      b. contribute to certain disorders
      c. lead to accidents and injuries
      d. all of the above

_______ **13.** According to the stress model, an emotional response can lead to a
      a. physical response
      b. positive consequence
      c. different interpretation of the situation
      d. new situation

_______ **14.** You can change the way you interpret a situation by
      a. eliminating some stressors
      b. using relaxation techniques
      c. using selective awareness
      d. doing physical exercise

_______ **15.** Maria has a test tomorrow. The thought of taking the test is causing her so much stress that she cannot concentrate on studying. Maria decides to sit quietly and close her eyes. She concentrates on her breathing and every time she breathes out, she thinks the word *calm*. Maria is using
      a. progressive relaxation   c. meditation
      b. autogenic training   d. imagery

_______ **16.** Paul just had an argument with his friend. Paul is feeling angry and stressed. He tries to use progressive relaxation, but it does not seem to be working this time. Paul's muscles are too tense. The best thing for Paul to try is
      a. selective awareness   c. eliminating stressors
      b. imagery   d. physical exercise

_______ **17.** The negative consequences of stress can be prevented by
      a. exercising regularly   c. eating a balanced diet
      b. using relaxation techniques   d. all of the above

_______ **18.** An effective way to manage stress is to
      a. talk to people you can trust
      b. use alcohol or drugs
      c. sleep
      d. all of the above

_______ **19.** A support group that a person can use to help manage stress is
      a. friends and family   c. a school counselor
      b. a minister, priest, or rabbi   d. all of the above

Part III ....

Listed below are the steps of the stress model you studied. Identify each step as either Step 1, Step 2, Step 3, Step 4, or Step 5 by putting the appropriate number in front of each step.

_______ **20.** The negative consequences

_______ **21.** Your emotional response

_______ **22.** Your new or potentially unpleasant situation

_______ **23.** Your physical response

_______ **24.** You interpret the situation as threatening

Part IV ....

Answer the question in the space provided.

25. Your friend Lisa is feeling very stressed. She has a test to study for, a paper due that must be typed, and a speech to write. In addition to the schoolwork, Lisa must do the supper dishes and practice the piano. She just received a phone call to baby-sit this evening. Lisa doesn't feel she can say no to the baby-sitting, but she also doesn't feel she has enough time to do all that she must. What would you advise Lisa to do to help relieve her stress?

____

____

____

____

____

____

Chapter 10

Coping With Loss
Chapter Test

Part I

Match the terms on the left with the definitions on the right.

_____ **1.** cremation

_____ **2.** funeral

_____ **3.** grief

_____ **4.** hospice

_____ **5.** living will

_____ **6.** terminal illness

_____ **7.** will

a. a place for terminally ill people to live that offers medical care and counseling for the patient and counseling for the family

b. a legal document describing what should be done with a person's possessions after the person's death

c. the complete reduction of a body to ashes by intense heat

d. a ceremony at which others pay respect to the person who died

e. a deep feeling of distress caused by a loss, especially through death

f. a document expressing a terminally ill person's wish not to have medical equipment used to prolong his or her life when there is no hope for meaningful recovery

g. an illness or disorder that leads ultimately to death

Part II

Write the letter of the correct answer in the blank.

_____ **8.** Death
    a. occurs when the lungs and heart cease to function
    b. is a natural part of life
    c. is always sudden
    d. all of the above

_____ **9.** Elana has learned that her grandfather has advanced cancer and has about three months to live. Her first reaction to this news will most likely be
    a. depression
    b. anger
    c. shock and denial
    d. acceptance

_____ **10.** Maggie has been living with a terminal illness for almost a year now. Just recently, she has called her lawyer to make a will and has talked to her family about how she would like her funeral arranged. In facing death, Maggie is in the stage known as
    a. acceptance
    b. bargaining
    c. depression
    d. denial

______ **11.** A friend of yours has been diagnosed with AIDS. He told you that his disease is going to go into permanent remission because now he is going to go to church and take time to help people who are needy. Your friend is in the stage known as

a. depression
b. denial

c. bargaining
d. acceptance

______ **12.** Jeremy has just found out he has leukemia. He told you he knows that this isn't true and that the doctor received the wrong laboratory report. You can help Jeremy through this stage by

a. telling him the doctors are right and he is just going to have to face the facts
b. listening to what Jeremy has to say
c. agreeing with what Jeremy is saying
d. telling Jeremy not to worry because you just read that scientists have found a cure for leukemia

______ **13.** Dying people need and want

a. some control over what is happening to them
b. a supportive group of family and friends
c. to die with dignity
d. all of the above

______ **14.** Hospice care is a choice that dying people have available. Some people choose hospice care because hospices

a. often provide care in the patient's own home
b. freely administer medications for pain control
c. allow family visitations without age or hour restrictions
d. all of the above

______ **15.** A living will

a. expresses a person's legal right to take his or her life
b. allows a person to refuse treatment to continue his or her life if there is no hope for meaningful recovery
c. allows the patient's family to decide what medical treatment should be given
d. all of the above

______ **16.** Angela's grandmother is in the hospital with a terminal illness. The grandmother tells Angela that she knows she doesn't have long to live and that she is tired of the "cold" feeling of the hospital. The grandmother also tells Angela that she is tired of all the shots, blood tests, and intravenous fluids. She doesn't want to keep living this way, but she doesn't know what to do. Angela might help her grandmother by

a. encouraging her to talk about all the things that are making her sad and depressed
b. helping her find out more about hospice care
c. helping her find out more about a living will
d. all of the above

______ **17.** Memorial services

a. always have the body of the deceased person present
b. are formal religious services
c. help people accept the finality of death
d. all of the above

_______ **18.** A funeral is a service
       a. that is usually religious in nature
       b. in which the body of the deceased person is present
       c. that enables friends to show support to the grieving family
       d. all of the above

_______ **19.** Grief can be influenced by
       a. when the death occurred   c. how well you knew the person who died
       b. how the death occurred   d. all of the above

_______ **20.** The grieving process is experienced when there is a loss of a
       a. loved one through death   c. job you enjoyed
       b. love relationship   d. all of the above

_______ **21.** Aaron was very close to his father. Aaron's father was unexpectedly killed in a car accident. Aaron is grieving over the loss of his father. This grieving process could last
       a. just until after the funeral   c. for a couple of months
       b. for several weeks   d. for a year or more

_______ **22.** You could help Aaron through the grieving process by
       a. listening to him and letting him share his grief with you
       b. advising him on things he could do to make him put the loss of his father out of his mind
       c. assuring him that he'll get over the loss soon
       d. all of the above

_______ **23.** When you experience grief, it is important that you
       a. keep your feelings to yourself
       b. not cry—crying is a sign of weakness
       c. remember that recovery from a loss is a slow process
       d. all of the above

_______ **24.** Seeking help as you deal with grief is a sign of strength, not a sign of weakness. People who can help you through the grieving process include a
       a. good friend, teacher, or coach   c. priest, minister, or rabbi
       b. school counselor or therapist   d. all of the above

Part III

Answer the question in the space provided.

25. A close friend has just lost her grandmother. She tells you that although her grandmother was ill for some time, she was not expecting to feel so sad and lonely after her death. Your friend tells you that she feels angry at times and that at other times she feels depressed. What could you say to your friend?

____

____

____

____

NAME ______________________________ CLASS ______ DATE ______

Preventing Suicide
Chapter Test

Part I . . . .
Match the terms on the left with the definitions on the right.

_______ **1.** depression

_______ **2.** suicidal mindset

_______ **3.** suicide

_______ **4.** tunnel vision

a. the act of intentionally taking one's life

b. inability to see all options available

c. a state of feeling sad and hopeless

d. the feeling that suicide is the only solution to the problems of living

Part II . . . .
Write the letter of the correct answer in the blank.

_______ **5.** People may think about taking their own life when they feel
   a. hopeless
   b. constant pain
   c. isolated or lonely
   d. all of the above

_______ **6.** Suicide among teenagers is
   a. on the decline
   b. a leading cause of death
   c. completely understood
   d. all of the above

_______ **7.** A possible reason why a teenager might want to commit suicide is that he or she
   a. lives in a dysfunctional family and may have experienced physical, mental, or sexual abuse
   b. has low self-esteem
   c. has no support system of family or friends
   d. all of the above

_______ **8.** Most teenagers who commit suicide
   a. do so because they want to be glamorous or seem like a mythic figure
   b. do so for trivial reasons
   c. do not really want to die
   d. have examined all other options and found there is no alternative

_______ **9.** You notice that your friend Robert has been feeling down lately and that his grades have been dropping. He has also joked with you a couple of times about suicide. You should
   a. ask Robert if he is thinking about suicide
   b. keep your thoughts about Robert to yourself
   c. avoid mentioning suicide
   d. try to make Robert feel better by telling him to "snap out of it"

_____ **10.** Warning signs of suicide might include
      a. direct statements about suicide
      b. inability to concentrate
      c. feelings of depression
      d. all of the above

_____ **11.** Some situations that might lead to suicidal thoughts or behavior include
      a. the loss of a relationship
      b. quitting taking drugs
      c. a wanted pregnancy
      d. all of the above

_____ **12.** If you feel suicidal, the best thing to do is
      a. keep your thoughts to yourself
      b. confide in a friend, but make him or her promise not to tell anyone
      c. seek help from a trusted adult
      d. turn to drugs or alcohol to make you feel better

_____ **13.** There are several people you can contact if you need to get help for a suicidal friend. These people include
      a. a relative, such as an aunt
      b. a teacher
      c. a priest, minister, or rabbi
      d. all of the above

Part III ·

Write M on the line next to statements that are myths about suicide. Write F next to statements that are facts about suicide.

_____ **14.** Once a person is suicidal, he or she will always be suicidal.

_____ **15.** The tendency toward suicide is inherited and passed from parent to child.

_____ **16.** A suicide attempt is often a cry for help.

_____ **17.** Most people who commit suicide have talked about doing so before.

_____ **18.** All suicidal people are mentally ill.

_____ **19.** If someone talks about committing suicide while drunk or high, that person shouldn't be taken seriously.

Part IV ·

Listed below are some behaviors that may or may not be appropriate in helping a suicidal person. Place an *X* on the line in front of the behaviors that would be helpful.

______ **20.** Trust your feelings if you think a person is suicidal and ask him or her about suicide.

______ **21.** Dismiss the person's feelings as temporary or assume that he or she will get over them.

______ **22.** Leave the suicidal person alone to deal with his or her problems.

______ **23.** Let the suicidal person know you are listening and understanding what he or she is saying.

______ **24.** Get help for the suicidal person even if he or she makes you promise you will not do so.

Part V ·

Answer the question in the space provided.

25. Maria and Steve were talking about their friend Krista. Steve was telling Maria that he noticed that Krista seemed really depressed lately. Maria said that she noticed it as well. Krista had not cared to do much of anything lately. She had not even wanted to go to the movies. Steve told Maria that he thought it was strange that yesterday evening Krista called him and asked if he would take Shadow, her pet dog. What do you think Maria and Steve should do about Krista, if anything? Why?

Chapter 12

The Use, Misuse, and Abuse of Drugs
Chapter Test

Part I

Match the terms on the left with the definitions on the right.

_____ **1.** analgesic

_____ **2.** drug

_____ **3.** drug abuse

_____ **4.** drug misuse

_____ **5.** drug use

_____ **6.** medicine

_____ **7.** sedative

_____ **8.** stimulant

a. taking a medicine exactly as directed

b. improper use of a medicine

c. a medicine that relieves pain

d. a substance that causes a physical or emotional change in a person

e. a drug that speeds up body functions

f. use of a legal drug for nonmedical reasons or any use of an illegal drug

g. a drug that slows down body functions and causes sleepiness

h. a substance that is used to treat an illness or ailment

Part II

Write the letter of the correct answer in the blank.

_____ **9.** Which of the following is a problem of living in a drug-oriented society?

    a. Advertisements provide too much information on drugs.
    b. Most over-the-counter drugs are not effective.
    c. Many people think drugs can solve all their problems.
    d. Drugs treat the symptoms, not the disease.

_____ **10.** Which of the following is the main message we receive from drug advertising?

    a. If we take a drug, we'll feel better.
    b. Drugs should be used only rarely.
    c. We don't need to seek the advice of a doctor.
    d. all the above

_____ **11.** Headaches are often caused by stress. Which of the following usually helps relieve stress?

    a. sedatives
    b. physical exercise
    c. coffee or tea
    d. a small alcoholic drink

_______ **12.** Peter broke his arm playing football. The doctor wrote a prescription for a painkiller. The prescription said to take one tablet every four hours as needed for pain. Peter only took two tablets—one after he got home from having his arm set and another four hours later. Those were the only times his arm hurt. Peter

    a. abused the painkillers
    b. used the painkillers correctly
    c. misused the painkillers
    d. became addicted to the painkillers

_______ **13.** Steve, Peter's brother, had a terrible headache. He looked in the medicine cabinet for some aspirin. He found Peter's prescription painkillers. Steve decided to take one tablet of the painkiller instead of the aspirin. Steve

    a. abused the drug
    b. misused the drug
    c. used a drug correctly
    d. became addicted to a drug

_______ **14.** Dana had not been able to sleep. She started taking an over-the-counter medication to help her sleep. Although the directions said to take two pills, Dana took three pills, thinking that an extra pill would help her sleep that much better. Dana

    a. misused the drug
    b. abused the drug
    c. become addicted to the drug
    d. all of the above

_______ **15.** Taking a drug is safest when it is

    a. bought
    b. taken as prescribed
    c. drunk as a tea
    d. used for minor illnesses

_______ **16.** The effects of a medicine can be influenced by whether

    a. it was taken with a lot of water
    b. the patient had eaten before taking it
    c. it was sold over-the-counter
    d. it was in a safety bottle

_______ **17.** Dewayne had a bad cold. He decided to take an over-the-counter medication to help relieve his cold symptoms. After he took the medication, he began to feel very sleepy. This feeling of sleepiness is most likely due to

    a. side effects of the drug
    b. misuse of the drug
    c. interactions among drugs
    d. allergy

Part III ·

Use the prescription label shown below to answer the questions. Write your answers in the spaces provided.

Home Town Pharmacy   **200 Alameda Street**
Home Town, CA   **619-555-9000**

RX 1257362   Dr. Takamura   10/15/96

Refills: 0

Drug Exp: 10/97

Smith, Pamela

Take one tablet 4 times daily for 10 days.

28 Penicillin VK   TAB 500mg

Best if medication is taken on an empty stomach.

18. When was the prescription filled? _______________________________________

19. Who is the prescription for? ____

20. Who wrote the prescription? ____

21. Who filled the prescription? ____

22. How should the medication be taken? ___________________________________

23. What is the name of the medication? ___________________________________

24. What is the dosage of the medication? __________________________________

25. When does the medication expire? _____________________________________

Chapter 13

Alcohol: A Dangerous Drug

Chapter Test

Part I

Match the terms on the left with the definitions on the right.

_____ **1.** alcoholism

_____ **2.** cirrhosis

_____ **3.** hangover

_____ **4.** hepatitis

_____ **5.** intoxication

_____ **6.** withdrawal

a. being affected by alcohol

b. the process of discontinuing a drug to which the body has become addicted

c. inflammation of the liver

d. uncomfortable physical effects brought on by alcohol use

e. condition in which healthy liver cells are replaced by scar tissue

f. the state of being psychologically and physically addicted to alcohol

Part II

Write the letter of the best answer in the blank.

_____ **7.** Alcohol is a dangerous drug because it
  a. is absorbed in the bloodstream
  b. travels to the brain
  c. can change the way the body functions
  d. gives some people a sense of excitement

_____ **8.** Jack drank three bottles of beer in two hours. This is enough alcohol to
  a. make him feel relaxed   c. affect his coordination
  b. impair his vision   d. all of the above

_____ **9.** Long-term alcohol abuse can lead to
  a. impaired judgment
  b. irreversible memory damage
  c. irreversible hearing damage
  d. all of the above

_____ **10.** Long-term alcohol abuse can damage the
  a. liver   c. hearing
  b. lungs   d. all of the above

_____ **11.** Jennifer has been having arguments with her parents about her boyfriend. Her grades at school have also been dropping. Jennifer is upset and feeling depressed. She goes to a party and begins to drink. Jennifer is most likely drinking
  a. to forget her problems   c. for excitement
  b. to be glamorous   d. to feel relaxed

_______ **12.** Which of the following is a good reason to drink?

    a. to feel relaxed
    b. to be more social
    c. to get high
    d. none the above

_______ **13.** A myth concerning alcohol is

    a. not everyone shows the effects of alcohol in the same way
    b. you can't get as drunk on wine as you can on hard liquor
    c. it is dangerous to drive a car after drinking one bottle of beer
    d. all of the above

_______ **14.** Marco is at a party. His friend, Bill, offers him a glass of whiskey. Marco doesn't want to drink because he drove to the party. He also knows that his parents do not want him to drink. Marco makes a responsible decision by deciding

    a. not to drink any alcohol
    b. to have only one glass of whiskey
    c. to drink only beer instead of hard liquor
    d. to drink as much as he wants but get a ride home with someone else instead of driving home

_______ **15.** A person who cannot drink alcohol in moderation is said to be

    a. dependent upon alcohol
    b. abusing alcohol
    c. addicted to alcohol
    d. experiencing withdrawal from alcohol

_______ **16.** A person who has to have a regular "fix" of alcohol is in the final phase of alcoholism, which is known as

    a. withdrawal   c. dependency
    b. alcohol syndrome   d. addiction

_______ **17.** Kathy has been doing poorly in school. She has been drinking every day for several months. She can't wait until school is over to go home to have a drink. It seems as if she is always thinking about a drink. Which of the following describes Kathy?

    a. She is physically addicted to alcohol.
    b. She is dependent upon alcohol.
    c. She is in withdrawal.
    d. She is a codependent.

_______ **18.** People who abuse alcohol most likely

    a. do poorly in school or at their job
    b. engage in risky behavior
    c. abuse their family
    d. all of the above

_____ **19.** A sign of alcohol abuse is
  a. improved relationships   c. irritability
  b. seizures   d. all of the above

_____ **20.** Pregnant women who drink alcohol put their children at risk for fetal alcohol syndrome. Symptoms of this syndrome include
  a. low birth weight   c. mental retardation
  b. facial deformities   d. all of the above

_____ **21.** A parent's alcoholism can affect his or her children through
  a. physical abuse   c. emotional abuse
  b. mental abuse   d. all of the above

_____ **22.** Which of the following is true of alcoholism?
  a. It affects only the alcoholic.
  b. It is a mental illness.
  c. It can be treated successfully.
  d. all of the above

_____ **23.** Treatment for alcoholism includes
  a. admitting powerlessness over alcohol
  b. withdrawal
  c. inpatient or outpatient counseling
  d. all of the above

_____ **24.** Help for alcoholics and family members of alcoholics is available through
  a. Al-Anon   c. Alcoholics Anonymous
  b. hospital programs   d. all of the above

Part III

Answer the question in the space provided.

25. Becky and you went to a party together. Becky picked you up at your house. You both agreed to leave the party at 11:30 P.M. At 11:00 P.M. you went to find Becky. She was drinking. You noticed her speech was slurred and she had trouble standing. Would you ride with Becky? Why or why not? If you decided not to ride with Becky, what would you do to get home?

____

____

____

____

____

____

Chapter 14

Tobacco: Hazardous and Addictive

Chapter Test

Part I

Match the terms on the left with the definitions on the right.

_____ **1.** cancer

_____ **2.** carbon monoxide

_____ **3.** cardiovascular disease

_____ **4.** chronic bronchitis

_____ **5.** cilia

_____ **6.** emphysema

_____ **7.** mainstream smoke

_____ **8.** sidestream smoke

a. tiny hairs that line the bronchial tubes

b. smoke that is inhaled directly into the mouth and lungs through a cigar, pipe, or cigarette

c. a gas that is found in tobacco smoke and interferes with the blood's ability to carry oxygen

d. a disease caused by cells that have lost normal growth controls and that invade and destroy healthy tissue

e. an inflammation of the bronchial tubes in the lungs and the production of excessive mucus

f. smoke that enters the environment from burning tobacco

g. disease of the heart and blood vessels

h. a disease in which the air sacs of the lungs are ruptured or torn

Part II

Write the letter of the correct answer in the blank.

_____ **9.** The chemical in tobacco that is a psychoactive substance and is addictive is

    a. tar

    b. nicotine

    c. carbon monoxide

    d. nitrogen dioxide

_____ **10.** The chemical in tobacco smoke that is made up of solid particles that contribute to the destruction of cilia and respiratory disease is

    a. carbon monoxide

    b. ammonia

    c. tar

    d. nicotine

_____ **11.** Which of the following is *not* true of lung cancer?

    a. It causes over 120,000 deaths per year.

    b. It is the most common cause of cancer deaths among American women.

    c. The risk of developing it can be greatly reduced by not smoking or breathing smoke.

    d. Its connection to cigarette smoking is unclear.

_____ **12.** Smoking is directly related to and can increase one's risk for

    a. heart attack

    b. kidney cancer

    c. stroke

    d. all of the above

______ **13.** Jason's father has been smoking for many years. His lungs have trouble absorbing oxygen from the air and pushing out carbon dioxide. As a result, Jason's father is always short of breath. Jason's father most likely has

    a. bronchitis   c. lung cancer
    b. emphysema   d. respiratory failure

______ **14.** The most dangerous use of tobacco is

    a. pipe smoking   c. cigarette smoking
    b. tobacco chewing d. breathing others' smoke

______ **15.** Using smokeless tobacco—chewing tobacco and snuff—can put one at greater risk of

    a. emphysema   c. mouth cancer
    b. lung cancer   d. all of the above

______ **16.** The tobacco smoke that rises from a lit pipe is called

    a. passive smoke   c. mainstream smoke
    b. sidestream smoke d. filtered smoke

______ **17.** Angela does *not* smoke. However, she works in an office where several co-workers smoke cigarettes all day long. Which of the following is *not* true of Angela?

    a. She would be no worse off if she herself smoked.
    b. She is a passive smoker.
    c. She is at risk for lung cancer.
    d. She is subject to sidestream smoke.

______ **18.** Katya has just found out she is pregnant. She and her husband, Jeff, smoke. They would be wise to stop smoking because

    a. smoking can cause a miscarriage
    b. the developing fetus could be born too early if Katya continued to smoke
    c. even though Katya may stop smoking, the smoke from Jeff's cigarettes could affect the baby
    d. all of the above

______ **19.** Rodger quit smoking five years ago. His chances of getting lung cancer are now

    a. decreased by 50%
    b. decreased by 25%
    c. decreased by 75%
    d. as low as they would be if he had never smoked

______ **20.** Which of the following is least likely to encourage a young person to quit smoking?

    a. Friends who don't smoke
    b. A desire to participate in sports
    c. Knowledge about the health consequences of smoking
    d. Parents who smoke but tell their children not to smoke

_____ **21.** At first, Ellen thought it was glamorous to smoke. But now she's tired of being short of breath and coughing every morning. If she quits, she will

    a. stop coughing and feel better
    b. enable the cilia in her bronchial tubes to repair themselves
    c. immediately reduce her risk for lung and other cancers
    d. all of the above

_____ **22.** Paula works in a high-stress job. She and most of her co-workers smoke. It will be particularly hard for her to quit because

    a. cigarette smoking leads to the use of other drugs.
    b. her stress cannot be handled in other ways.
    c. she may have little support from the people she is with all day.
    d. she will have to breathe sidestream smoke.

_____ **23.** Which of the following would probably *not* help Paula stop successfully?

    a. Spontaneously throwing away her cigarettes one day at work
    b. Gradually cutting down the number of cigarettes she smokes
    c. Talking with her doctor about a nicotine patch
    d. Waiting until she is on vacation to stop smoking

Part III

Answer the question in the space provided.

24. Most doctors' offices and hospitals have adopted a nonsmoking policy. How might they justify this policy?

____

____

____

____

____

25. Give three reasons a pregnant woman should not smoke.

____

____

____

____

Chapter 15

Other Drugs of Abuse

Chapter Test

Part I

Match the definitions on the right with the terms on the left.

______ **1.** addicted

______ **2.** dependent

______ **3.** drug abuse

______ **4.** hallucinogen

______ **5.** inhalant

______ **6.** narcotic

______ **7.** psychoactive drug

______ **8.** stimulant

______ **9.** withdrawal

a. the use of a legal drug for nonmedical reasons or an illegal drug for any reason

b. a physical process in which the body cannot function without a certain substance

c. a drug that affects a person's mood and behavior

d. being controlled by a psychological or physical desire for a psychoactive drug

e. the body's reaction when it does not receive a drug it depends on

f. a drug that causes alertness and speeds up the activity of the body

g. a drug that distorts a person's senses

h. a chemical that produces strong psychoactive effects when inhaled

i. a drug with strong pain-relieving and psychoactive properties that is made from the opium plant

Part II

Write the letter of the correct answer in the blank.

______ **10.** Terry has a difficult job. Her manager wants her to do everything perfectly the first time. Terry's family members are demanding, too, and want her to help around the house. To relax from all the stress, Terry takes drugs every Friday night. Terry's major problem is her

a. difficult job

b. drug abuse

c. unreasonable manager

d. demanding family

______ **11.** Ken takes drugs every day. To support his drug habit, he shoplifts from department stores and steals from people's houses. Which phrase describes Ken best?

a. Drug abuser who hurts department stores

b. Drug abuser who hurts all society

c. Drug abuser who hurts some homeowners

d. Drug abuser who hurts himself

_____ **12.** Jack started using cocaine just to fit in with his friends. Soon, Jack found out that he needed a larger dose of the drug in order to experience the same effect, or high. If Jack did not take a higher dosage, he became very restless and irritable. Which of the following has Jack developed?

a. A tolerance for cocaine   c. A mental illness
b. Withdrawal symptoms   d. Signs of recovery

_____ **13.** A person who is most likely to resist peer pressure to try drugs usually has which of the following characteristics?

a. High self-esteem
b. Depression
c. A need to be liked by others
d. All of the above

_____ **14.** The first step in drug addiction is

a. psychological dependence   c. withdrawal
b. tolerance   d. physical dependence

_____ **15.** People who use psychoactive drugs often experience

a. enhanced judgment   c. loss of control
b. increased concentration   d. all of the above

_____ **16.** Crack differs from cocaine in that crack

a. is less addictive
b. affects the brain more quickly
c. is inhaled instead of smoked
d. all of the above

_____ **17.** Crack and cocaine are dangerous because they

a. are addictive   c. can be fatal
b. can cause violent behavior   d. all of the above

_____ **18.** Rose was spray painting an art project in an enclosed garage. Soon, Rose noticed that she was feeling lightheaded, dizzy, and nauseated. What should Rose do?

a. Stop spray painting immediately and step outside
b. Open the garage doors and keep on painting
c. Finish the painting but don't use the paint again
d. Complain to the paint manufacturer about a defective product

_____ **19.** Which of the following is true of heroin?

a. An overdose with heroin is unlikely.
b. It is always sold in pure form.
c. Users are at risk for hepatitis and AIDS.
d. Users can inject heroin safely for years.

_____ **20.** A drug that is used for medical purposes but that can also be easily abused is

a. barbiturates   c. cocaine
b. PCP   d. heroin

_____ **21.** Sarah's boyfriend, Joe, tells her he is thinking of taking steroids. Sarah should tell Joe
  - a. it is okay since many athletes take steroids
  - b. it is a great idea since she likes "big, strong, muscular" men
  - c. steroids can cause more harm than good
  - d. steroids will help him improve his performance on the football team

_____ **22.** When overcoming a drug addiction, a person must go through
  - a. withdrawal
  - b. a self-help program
  - c. an inpatient program
  - d. group therapy

_____ **23.** A person who wants to seek treatment for drug dependency should realize that
  - a. he or she does not have to do it alone
  - b. there is no such thing as a fully recovered addict
  - c. he or she must overcome the psychological reasons for drug abuse
  - d. all of the above

_____ **24.** Tom's parents are going through a divorce. Tom is feeling angry, frustrated, sad, and depressed. One of Tom's friends offers him some pills, telling him that the pills would make him feel better. What should Tom do?
  - a. Take the pills
  - b. Talk to an adult he feels he can confide in
  - c. Call the National Drug Information and Referral Line
  - d. all of the above

Part III . . . .

Answer the question in the space provided.

25. You are at a party and notice that your friend is sniffing some white powder from a tiny spoon. You confront your friend and he tells you the white powder is cocaine. He offers you some and tells you it is relatively harmless and makes you feel good. You refuse and tell him that you do not want to become addicted to drugs. He tells you that cocaine is not addictive and that he has been using it for over a year and can quit any time he wants. What concerns might you have for your friend, and what would you do about these concerns?

____

____

____

____

____

____

____

Chapter 16

Reproduction and the Early Years of Life
Chapter Test

Part I

Match the terms on the left with the definitions on the right.

_____ **1.** egg

_____ **2.** embryo

_____ **3.** fertilization

_____ **4.** fetus

_____ **5.** ovaries

_____ **6.** ovulation

_____ **7.** placenta

_____ **8.** semen

_____ **9.** sperm

_____ **10.** testes

a. male reproductive cell

b. female reproductive cell

c. male reproductive structures that produce sperm

d. sperm plus protective fluids

e. the union of a sperm and an egg

f. female reproductive structures that produce eggs

g. the release of an egg

h. the structure that enables an embryo to obtain nutrients from its mother

i. developing individual from the ninth week of pregnancy until birth

j. a fertilized egg after it has attached itself to the wall of the uterus

Part II

Write the letter of the correct answer on the line provided.

_____ **11.** A function of the testes is to

    a. make estrogen

    b. make sperm

    c. deliver sperm to the outside of the body

    d. add fluid to sperm

_____ **12.** Testosterone is a hormone that is

    a. responsible for male sex characteristics

    b. necessary for sperm production

    c. produced by the testes

    d. all of the above

_____ **13.** The last organ that the sperm pass through before leaving the body is the

    a. vas deferens

    b. epididymis

    c. penis

    d. prostate gland

_____ **14.** The process by which sperm leave the body is called

    a. ejaculation

    b. fertilization

    c. circumcision

    d. contraction

_____ **15.** Once inside a woman's body, sperm
  a. travel up the fallopian tubes
  b. get trapped in mucus and die
  c. release enzymes that break down the layer of cells surrounding the egg
  d. all of the above

_____ **16.** A function of the uterus is to
  a. produce an egg
  b. provide shelter and nourishment for the developing egg
  c. provide nourishment for the baby after birth
  d. all of the above

_____ **17.** In order for an egg to unite with a sperm, the egg
  a. cannot have been released more than 24 hours ago
  b. must be in the ovary
  c. must be in the uterus
  d. all of the above

_____ **18.** The monthly changes the uterus undergoes are called the
  a. menstrual syndrome   c. menstrual period
  b. menstrual fluid   d. menstrual cycle

_____ **19.** Monthly changes in the uterus include
  a. thickening of the lining   c. shedding of the lining
  b. lining breaking down   d. all of the above

_____ **20.** A breast self-exam should be done
  a. every month   c. to check for discharge from nipples
  b. to check for lumps   d. all of the above

_____ **21.** A testicular self-exam should be done monthly to check for
  a. testicular torsion   c. inguinal hernia
  b. testicular cancer   d. all of the above

_____ **22.** Substances that can pass from the mother to the placenta include
  a. over-the-counter medications
  b. alcohol
  c. chemicals from cigarette smoke
  d. all of the above

_____ **23.** The first stage of labor involves
  a. the baby being born
  b. contractions that dilate, or widen, the cervix
  c. the placenta being expelled, or released, from the uterus
  d. all of the above

_______ **24.** Childhood experiences may be happy or painful. A person might successfully deal with these experiences by

    a. making the most of the positive experiences
    b. minimizing the effects of negative experiences
    c. using the process known as self-talk
    d. all of the above

Part III ·

Number the stages of the menstrual cycle in the order they occur.

_______ **25.** The lining of the uterus thickens.

_______ **26.** The egg is not fertilized in the fallopian tube.

_______ **27.** An ovary releases an egg.

_______ **28.** Menstrual fluid is released from the body.

_______ **29.** The thickened uterine lining breaks down.

Part IV ·

Answer the question in the space provided.

30. How do you think childhood experiences affect a person's self-esteem?

____

____

____

____

____

____

____

____

____

Chapter 17

Adolescence: Relationships and Responsibilities

Chapter Test

Part I

Match the definitions on the right with the correct terms on the left.

_____ **1.** active listening

_____ **2.** emotional intimacy

_____ **3.** empathy

_____ **4.** heterosexuals

_____ **5.** homosexuals

_____ **6.** mixed message

_____ **7.** nonverbal communication

_____ **8.** puberty

_____ **9.** sexual abstinence

_____ **10.** sexual intimacy

a. the period of physical development during which people become able to reproduce

b. body language, such as eye contact, facial expressions, and body position, that sends a message

c. the process of hearing the words of the speaker and clarifying anything that is confusing

d. a type of communication in which verbal and nonverbal messages do not match

e. people who are sexually attracted to those of the same sex

f. the ability to understand another person's feelings

g. sharing thoughts and feelings and learning to trust one another

h. people who are sexually attracted to those of the opposite sex

i. breast and genital touching and sexual intercourse

j. refraining from sexual intimacy

Part II

Write the letter of the correct answer in the blank.

_____ **11.** Ryan was afraid of being turned down, but he asked Kim to the fall dance anyway. Kim told him she wasn't able to go with him because she had already accepted an invitation from Bob. Kim told Ryan that perhaps they could go out another time. Ryan was disappointed. But as he thought about Kim's response, he decided Kim didn't say no because she didn't like him, but because she already had a date. Ryan decided to call and ask Linda to the dance. Which statement best describes the situation?

    a. Kim is giving mixed messages.
    b. Ryan should use the RESPECT method of resolving conflicts.
    c. Kim is playing hard to get.
    d. Ryan is growing emotionally and socially.

_____ **12.** Marylu and Kirsten had a disagreement about what to do Saturday night. Marylu wanted to go to the movies. Kirsten wanted to go to a party. Both left angry. The next afternoon, Marylu called Kirsten. Marylu wanted to resolve this conflict. How could she best do this?

    a. Use "you" messages.
    b. Communicate at an information-giving level.
    c. Separate the issue of friendship from what she wanted to do.
    d. Use "I" messages.

______ **13.** It was the second time Jeff and Theresa went out on a date. Jeff told Theresa how much he loved her and that he wanted to show her he meant this by making love to her. Theresa looked Jeff directly in the eyes and told him that she was not ready to become sexually intimate. Jeff insisted that she really wanted to but was playing hard to get. Which statement best represents the type of communication that took place between Jeff and Theresa?

    a. Jeff is using active-listening skills.
    b. Jeff was sending mixed messages.
    c. Theresa was verbally and nonverbally resisting pressure.
    d. Theresa was using "you" messages.

______ **14.** Vivian has just transferred to a new school. She wants to make new friends. What is the best way for her to do so?

    a. Find out who the popular students are and make friends with them
    b. Join a club that does things she likes to do
    c. Wait until someone notices her and tries to make friends with her
    d. Consider only another person who is shy and always alone as the best person to becomes friends with

______ **15.** Karen just told Tony that she did not want to date him any longer. Tony is devastated by this decision. He should

    a. be good to himself and indulge in something he likes to do
    b. brood about what he did or did not do to make the relationship fail
    c. keep to himself for several weeks until he gets over the breakup
    d. insist on talking to Karen, thinking she was probably upset about something and didn't really mean it

______ **16.** Tim and Ashley have been dating steadily for six months. They both are considering becoming sexually intimate. Which of the following statements represents sound reasoning?

    a. The best way to get to know someone is through sexual intimacy.
    b. They should seriously consider whether they are too young for the commitment sexual intimacy would require.
    c. Sexual intimacy will help them reach a higher level of emotional intimacy.
    d. The best way for them to express their love for one another is through sexual intimacy.

______ **17.** If your boyfriend or girlfriend tries to pressure you into sexual intimacy and you don't feel you want to be intimate, you should

    a. feel guilty if you say no
    b. remember you have the right to refuse sexual intimacy at anytime for any reason
    c. keep in mind that if you say no you may lose your boyfriend or girlfriend
    d. wonder if something is wrong with you

Part III ·

Complete the chart below by filling in the spaces with the appropriate changes.

PHYSICAL CHANGES OCCURRING AT PUBERTY	
MALE	**FEMALE**
Grow taller	Grow taller
Acne	Acne
18.	——
19.	——
Underarm hair; perspiration	Underarm hair; perspiration
Shoulders broaden; muscles develop	**20.**
21.	**22.**
23.	**24.**
Pubic hair	Pubic hair

Part IV ·

Answer the question in the space provided.

25. Why is it a good idea to decide before dating how intimate you wish to become and to think about how to resist pressure to go beyond the level of intimacy with which you feel comfortable?

____

____

____

____

____

____

____

____

Chapter 18

Adulthood, Marriage, and Parenthood
Chapter Test

Part I

Match the definitions on the right with the terms on the left.

_____ **1.** Alzheimer's disease

_____ **2.** contraception

_____ **3.** divorce

_____ **4.** emotional maturity

_____ **5.** middle adulthood

_____ **6.** older adulthood

_____ **7.** Parkinson's disease

_____ **8.** physical maturity

_____ **9.** separation

_____ **10.** young adulthood

a. period of adulthood between the ages of 20 and 40

b. fully developed and fully grown

c. married couple living apart for a period of time

d. an incurable disease that is characterized by a gradual loss of muscle function

e. period of adulthood that begins at age 65

f. the capacity to act independently, responsibly, and unselfishly

g. an incurable illness characterized by a gradual and permanent loss of memory

h. period of adulthood between the ages of 41 and 65

i. legal end of a marriage

j. a device or method that prevents fertilization or implantation of a woman's egg

Part II

Write the letter of the correct answer in the blank.

_____ **11.** It is during middle adulthood that most people

    a. reach emotional maturity
    b. begin to enjoy themselves because some major responsibilities are completed
    c. decide to have children
    d. experience physical and mental deterioration

_____ **12.** Jessica's grandfather lives alone and still works. However, he has Parkinson's disease. He must walk with a cane and his hands shake. He told Jessica that he is concerned about what would happen if he fell during the night and couldn't get up. Jessica's grandfather is concerned about

    a. becoming a burden to his family
    b. appropriate housing
    c. his physical well-being
    d. forced retirement

_______ **13.** Peter's grandmother has Alzheimer's disease. His grandfather has been taking care of her, but he is finding this task to be more and more difficult as his grandmother's condition worsens. Peter's grandmother does not recognize family members, often gets violent, and has lost bladder control. Peter's grandmother might get the best care by

    a. having a visiting nurse come three days a week
    b. moving in with Peter's family
    c. moving to a retirement community
    d. moving into a nursing home

_______ **14.** During young adulthood, you most likely will confront issues of

    a. career
    b. retirement
    c. death
    d. all of the above

_______ **15.** The best reason for two people to marry is

    a. they love and respect each other
    b. they want to have children
    c. their combined incomes will give them better financial security
    d. they don't want to spend their lives alone

_______ **16.** A successful marriage depends on the partners being

    a. self-sufficient
    b. emotionally secure
    c. financially secure
    d. certain of their views

_______ **17.** Bill and Michelle are 19 years old. They will be graduating from high school in two months. Michelle just found out she is pregnant. Bill and Michelle decide to get married. A difficulty they probably face is

    a. financial support
    b. limited career choices
    c. giving up a social life
    d. all of the above

_______ **18.** The most important key to being a good parent is

    a. being able to support your children financially
    b. enforcing strict discipline
    c. being emotionally mature
    d. taking responsibility for your children's education

Part III

Identify the following statements as myths or facts concerning aging. If the statement is a myth, write M on the line provided. If the statement is a fact, write F.

_______ **19.** Most older people live in nursing homes.

_______ **20.** Older people need to stop exercising and rest more.

_______ **21.** Older people do not have trouble learning new things.

_______ **22.** Most elderly people are healthy and physically active.

_______ **23.** Older people cannot take care of themselves.

_______ **24.** An older adult is more likely to develop heart disease or cancer than a young adult.

Part IV

Answer the question in the space provided.

25. What lifestyle choices can you make now that will influence how healthy you will remain as you grow older? How will each choice influence your health?

____

____

____

____

____

____

____

____

____

Chapter 19

Families

Chapter Test

Part I

Match the definitions on the right with the terms on the left.

_____ **1.** blended family

_____ **2.** couple family

_____ **3.** divorce

_____ **4.** dysfunctional family

_____ **5.** extended family

_____ **6.** nuclear family

_____ **7.** single-parent family

_____ **8.** stepparent

a. consists of a mother, father, and one or more children

b. a parent in a blended family who is not a child's biological parent

c. consists of relatives from outside the nuclear family living in the same home with the nuclear family

d. consists of only a husband and wife

e. a legal end to a marriage

f. results when a divorced parent remarries

g. family that does not fulfill the basic functions of a healthy family

h. consists of a mother or a father and one or more children

Part II

Write the letter of the correct answer in the blank.

_____ **9.** Jan is sick with the flu. Her mother has stayed home from work to be with her until Jan is well enough to return to school. Jan's mother is helping to fulfill the function of

    a. meeting basic physical needs
    b. providing emotional support
    c. providing structure
    d. meeting social needs

_____ **10.** Jason has two older brothers. One is married. The other is in college. Next month, Jason will start college, too. Jason's family is in the stage known as the

    a. beginning stage
    b. parenting stage
    c. empty-nest stage
    d. retirement stage

_____ **11.** Families of today differ from families in the 1950s and 1960s in that

    a. they are more likely to be nuclear families
    b. they are more likely to have a mother working outside the home
    c. they are better able to manage change
    d. they are not dysfunctional

_____ **12.** Families of today are smaller in size than families of the past because

    a. fewer parents rely on their children for financial support
    b. parents who own their own business hire other people to do the work
    c. raising children is very expensive
    d. all of the above

______ **13.** Usually in a divorce
   a. one parent is at fault
   b. the child or children are to blame
   c. there are several factors that contribute
   d. all of the above

______ **14.** Anita's parents have decided to get divorced. Anita cannot concentrate on her school work, finds it difficult to sleep, and has lost her appetite. Anita is reacting to the news about her parents' divorce by feeling
   a. angry
   b. depressed
   c. anxious
   d. guilty

______ **15.** You notice the change in Anita's behavior and ask her what is wrong. Anita tells you about her parents' divorce. You want to help Anita. What is one thing you should NOT do?
   a. Tell her not to worry because her parents may change their minds.
   b. Encourage her to become involved with a club at school.
   c. Suggest she talk with the school counselor or social worker.
   d. Let her know she can talk to you any time.

______ **16.** Paul's father has a drinking problem. He often criticizes Paul and tells him that he's the reason he drinks. Paul most likely
   a. is able to ignore his father's words
   b. has low self-esteem
   c. is able to get all the love he needs from his mother
   d. knows he is not to blame

______ **17.** What might Paul do to help himself deal with his family problems?
   a. Ignore the problems and wait until he is old enough to move out on his own.
   b. Move in with another family member or a friend.
   c. Seek counseling for his family or even just for himself.
   d. Become involved in a new hobby, sport, or school club.

Part III

Fill in the blank with the appropriate family characteristic.

18. Maria notices her sister's diary on the bed. Maria is tempted to read it, but she does not. Maria is showing

____

____

19. Billy failed his math test. He was feeling really bad. When he got home, his father noticed Billy's behavior. Billy's father looked him the eyes and said, "Billy, I can tell something is bothering you. Can we talk about it? I care about you and want to help if I can." Billy's dad was using

____

____

20. Billy tells his father about how hard he studied and how he failed the test anyway. He feels he'll never be able to understand math. Billy's dad puts his arm around Billy's shoulders and says, "Just because you did poorly on one test doesn't make you a failure. I'm proud of you for studying and trying your best. And I love you regardless of whether you get an A or an F on a test. Maybe I can help you with your homework." Billy's father is showing

____

21. Amanda's mother went back to work. Now on Saturday mornings Amanda's mother goes to the grocery store, her father washes the clothes, Amanda does the dishes, and her younger brother vacuums. Everyone in this family is showing the ability to

____

22. Julie's grandmother can no longer take care of herself. She moves in with Julie's family. Julie can't play her stereo as loud any more, and when Julie comes home from school, it is her job to get her grandmother a snack. Julie is glad to be able to help her grandmother. Julie is showing the ability to

____

Part IV . . . .

Read the paragraph below. Then answer the questions that follow.

Angela's father lost his job two months ago. Her mother has gone back to work full time to help meet the family's financial obligations. Angela is worried that if her father doesn't find a job soon, they may have to sell their home and move. Angela doesn't want to talk to her parents about her concerns because she feels they have enough on their minds right now. Not talking to her parents, however, has only added to the anxiety Angela is feeling because she has always been able to discuss any issue with them.

23. Would you classify Angela's family as healthy or dysfunctional? Explain.

____

____

____

24. What seems to be Angela's problem in the family? How can it be resolved?

____

____

____

25. Besides the answer you gave above, what alternative could Angela have?

____

____

____

Chapter 20

Preventing Abuse and Violence

Chapter Test

Part I

Match the definitions on the right with the correct terms on the left.

_____ **1.** acquaintance rape

_____ **2.** child abuse

_____ **3.** elder abuse

_____ **4.** emotional abuse

_____ **5.** homicide

_____ **6.** neglect

_____ **7.** physical abuse

_____ **8.** sexual abuse

_____ **9.** sexual assault

_____ **10.** spouse abuse

a. mistreatment of a child or adolescent

b. a violent crime that results in the death of another person

c. bodily harm inflicted on another person

d. the force or coercion of a person into sexual intercourse by an acquaintance or date

e. sexual behavior between an adult or adolescent and a nonconsenting person

f. failure of a parent or guardian to provide for the basic needs of a person in his or her charge

g. emotional mistreatment of another person

h. abuse of one's husband or wife

i. abuse of an elderly person

j. any sexual contact with a person without his or her consent

Part II

Write the letter of the correct answer in the blank.

_____ **11.** Most abused children and adolescents are abused by
    a. friends of the family
    b. strangers
    c. family members
    d. trusted caregivers

_____ **12.** Abused children most often come from homes in which
    a. one or both parents abuse drugs or alcohol
    b. a parent was also abused as a child
    c. a parent has personal problems
    d. all of the above

_____ **13.** A child who is emotionally abused will most likely
    a. have low self-esteem
    b. turn to others for emotional support
    c. report the abuse to authorities
    d. sexually abuse his or her children

_______ **14.** Many homicides can be avoided by preventing
    a. substance abuse
    b. gun possession
    c. violent arguments
    d. all of the above

_______ **15.** Many married women tolerate abuse from their husbands because the women
    a. deserve the abusive treatment
    b. like being abused
    c. feel they have no resources available
    d. may feel they deserve the abusive treatment

_______ **16.** Chrisann is on a date. Her date reaches over, forcefully pulls her next to him, and passionately kisses her. She pushes him away and says, "Stop." But he grabs her again and tries the same behavior. This is an example of
    a. sexual abuse   c. normal dating behavior
    b. acquaintance rape   d. sexual assault

_______ **17.** Most sexual assaults take place
    a. between an adult and a child
    b. in dark, deserted areas
    c. between two people who know each other
    d. because women encourage such behavior by the way they dress

_______ **18.** Joseph was telling Manuel that he couldn't wait for his date with Jennifer that night because this was going to be his "lucky" night. Joseph told Manuel that Jennifer had been hinting all week by the way she walked and by how she touched him that she wanted to have sexual intercourse with him. Considering Joseph's comments, what would be an appropriate response from Manuel?
    a. Remember that if Jennifer says no to sexual intercourse that is exactly what she means.
    b. There is a quiet, isolated place where they can park on the other side of town.
    c. Don't believe Jennifer if she changes her mind.
    d. Remember to be aggressive and in control.

_______ **19.** Ashley just got home from a date with a boy she has been seeing for three months. She calls you and is very upset. She tells you that her date forced her to have sexual intercourse with him after she repeatedly told him no. What would you tell Ashley?
    a. She asked for such behavior because she always flirts with her boyfriend.
    b. She should try to forget the incident because it is her word against his word.
    c. She should talk with her parents and inform the police.
    d. She should give him another chance.

_______ **20.** A young child is playing outside his home and a car drives by. Its occupants begin firing guns at the house next door. The child is hit by a bullet and is killed. This homicide is most likely related to
    a. sex   c. gang violence
    b. arguments   d. control of anger

______ **21.** Jason's parents have divorced. He doesn't see his father. His mother is always working to provide the physical needs for Jason and herself. Jason is approached and asked to become a member of a gang. What might be the main reason Jason would consider joining?

    a. A desire for status
    b. Lack of money
    c. Poor job prospects
    d. A sense of belonging to a family

______ **22.** Linda has had all she can take from Mary. Mary is always making fun of the way Linda looks and dresses. Linda told you that the next time Mary makes a comment about how she looks or dresses she is going to slap her in the face. What would you tell Mary?

    a. She should walk away and ignore Mary's comments.
    b. Slapping Mary would be a good idea; it would put her in her place.
    c. She should tell her older brother to take care of the problem.
    d. She is being oversensitive; Mary is only joking.

Part III

Read the paragraph below. Then answer the questions in the spaces provided.

As you change into your gym clothes in the locker room, you notice several welts across your friend's chest and back. When you ask her what happened, she tells you, "Nothing." When you pressure her further, she tells you that her boyfriend, who is 21 years old, was over the other night. No one else was home. He began to make sexual advances on her. When she kept telling him no, he became angry and took his belt off and hit her with it. This was not the first time he had hit her. You ask your friend if she told her parents. She says she can't because her boyfriend threatened to hurt her younger brother if she did.

23. What type(s) of abuse is your friend a victim of?

____

____

____

24. What would you recommend your friend do?

____

____

____

____

25. What would you do if this continued to happen and your friend took no action?

____

____

____

Infectious Diseases
Chapter Test

Part I

Match the terms on the left with the definitions on the right.

_____ **1.** antibiotic

_____ **2.** bacterium

_____ **3.** communicable disease

_____ **4.** immunization

_____ **5.** infection

_____ **6.** microorganism

_____ **7.** pathogen

_____ **8.** virus

a. a disease that is usually passed from one person to another

b. a single-celled microorganism that can cause disease

c. an agent that can cause a disease, such as the common cold or the flu

d. a tiny living being that is too small to be seen without the aid of a microscope

e. any agent that causes disease

f. a condition in which the body, or part of it, is invaded by a pathogen

g. an injection of a small amount of pathogen that will provide protection against the pathogen or the disease it causes

h. a medication that kills or limits the growth of bacteria

Part II

Write the letter of the correct answer in the blank.

_____ **9.** Which of the following is an infectious disease?

a. cancer
b. influenza
c. heart disease
d. all of the above

_____ **10.** Infectious diseases can be spread by

a. sneezing
b. kissing
c. sharing drinking glasses
d. all of the above

_____ **11.** Some infectious diseases can be spread by animals. One such disease is

a. ringworm
b. head lice
c. herpes simplex
d. all of the above

_____ **12.** Jack was picnicking with his family on a hot day. All the egg salad sandwiches, fried chicken, and apples got warm in the car, and everyone got food poisoning. The infection could probably have been prevented if

a. the hands and utensils had been kept clean
b. the food had been kept cold
c. the food had been cooked thoroughly
d. all of the above

______ **13.** A person can be said to have a disease when he or she
  a. has been exposed to a virus
  b. has been exposed to bacteria
  c. has signs and symptoms
  d. has been immunized

______ **14.** When a person has been infected with a cold pathogen, he or she may
  a. pass the disease on to someone else
  b. develop signs and symptoms
  c. be resistant to the pathogen
  d. all of the above

______ **15.** Suppose you put your fingers in your mouth without washing your hands. What is the first line of defense against any pathogens that you might swallow?
  a. white blood cells   c. T-cells
  b. stomach acid   d. antibodies

______ **16.** Immunity is an effective way to be protected against a disease. You can become immune to certain diseases by
  a. having had the disease once
  b. getting a vaccination for the disease
  c. having active memory cells for the disease
  d. all of the above

______ **17.** Which of the following is an infectious disease caused by a virus for which there is no vaccine?
  a. hepatitis B   c. common cold
  b. smallpox   d. all of the above

______ **18.** Which of the following is an infectious disease that can be cured by antibiotics?
  a. hepatitis A   c. chickenpox
  b. strep throat   d. all of the above

______ **19.** The chance of getting an infectious disease can be reduced by
  a. practicing good hygiene
  b. getting immunizations
  c. keeping your whole body healthy through exercise and a proper diet
  d. all of the above

Part III ·

Complete the chart below.

Infectious Diseases		
Disease	**Cause**	**Treatment or cure**
20. Influenza		rest and fluids
21. Strep throat	bacteria	
22. Measles	virus	
23. Common cold		rest and fluids
24. Mononucleosis		rest and fluids

Part IV ·

Answer the question in the space provided.

25. You are baby-sitting your 2-year-old brother, who has a cold. He has a runny nose, is sneezing, and is coughing. What steps can you take to reduce your chance of getting your brother's cold?

____

____

____

____

____

____

____

Sexually Transmitted Diseases

Chapter Test

Part I

Match the terms on the left with the definitions on the right.

_______ **1.** chancre

_______ **2.** vaginitis

_______ **3.** hepatitis

_______ **4.** infertility

_______ **5.** pelvic inflammatory disease

_______ **6.** scabies

_______ **7.** sexually transmitted disease

_______ **8.** nongonococcal urethritis

a. an inflammation of the vagina

b. an infection of the uterus and fallopian tubes

c. a disease that is passed from one person to another during sexual contact

d. an open sore that is filled with syphilis bacteria

e. an infection of the urethra that is caused by some agent other than gonorrhea

f. a skin condition that is caused by mites

g. an inflammation of the liver

h. the inability to have children

Part II

Write the letter of the correct answer in the blank.

_______ **9.** Gonorrhea is a sexually transmitted disease that

    a. is always fatal
    b. has symptoms of discharge in both men and women
    c. is caused by a virus
    d. all of the above

_______ **10.** Gonorrhea can infect the

    a. membranes of the penis and vagina
    b. throat
    c. rectum
    d. all of the above

_______ **11.** If untreated, gonorrhea

    a. will develop stronger symptoms
    b. always leads to infertility
    c. can be passed from mother to child during birth
    d. all of the above

_______ **12.** Pelvic inflammatory disease can
    a. affect both men and women
    b. lead to abdominal pain, fever, and infertility
    c. be detected by the presence of painful blisters
    d. all of the above

_______ **13.** Pelvic inflammatory disease can be caused by untreated
    a. gonorrhea   c. chlamydia
    b. bacterial infections   d. all of the above

_______ **14.** Chlamydia
    a. is often spread by people who don't know they have the disease
    b. can cause problems during a pregnancy
    c. can lead to infertility
    d. all of the above

_______ **15.** An STD that is characterized by painful blisters for which there is no cure is
    a. chlamydia   c. genital herpes
    b. genital warts   d. syphilis

_______ **16.** The secondary stage of syphilis is characterized by
    a. chancres   c. brain damage
    b. discharge   d. a rash

_______ **17.** The primary stage of syphilis is characterized by
    a. damage to nerves   c. a rash
    b. chancres   d. discharge

_______ **18.** An STD that is caused by a virus is
    a. chlamydia   c. trichomoniasis
    b. genital warts   d. vaginitis

_______ **19.** Vaginitis can be caused by
    a. chlamydia   c. trichomoniasis
    b. a yeast infection d. all of the above

_______ **20.** An STD caused by a parasite and characterized by intense itching is
    a. moniliasis   c. pubic lice
    b. chlamydia   d. all of the above

_______ **21.** You can decrease your chances of getting an STD by
    a. practicing sexual abstinence
    b. not using alcohol or drugs
    c. not sharing towels or clothing
    d. all of the above

_____ **22.** Showing affection for someone can be done safely by
    a. hugging   c. sexual intercourse
    b. French kissing   d. all of the above

_____ **23.** An STD that can be transmitted by ways other than sexual contact is
    a. genital herpes   c. scabies
    b. vaginitis   d. all of the above

_____ **24.** Paul thinks he might have an STD but is not sure. Which of the following should he *not* do?
    a. see his family doctor for a checkup
    b. wait to see if the symptoms go away
    c. go to the county health department for a test
    d. visit a public health clinic for a test

Part III

Answer the question in the space provided.

25. Angela tells you that about three weeks after she had intercourse with her boyfriend, Rob, she developed a vaginal discharge and mild pain in her lower abdomen. She asked Rob if he had any symptoms, but he said no. Angela wonders if she should just ignore the symptoms or try to treat the symptoms with over-the-counter medications. What would you advise Angela to do? Explain.

NAME _______________ CLASS ______ DATE ______

HIV Infection and AIDS

Chapter Test

Part I

Match the terms on the left with the definitions on the right.

______ **1.** abstinence

______ **2.** AIDS

______ **3.** condom

______ **4.** HIV

______ **5.** HIV-antibody test

______ **6.** HIV-positive

______ **7.** monogamy

______ **8.** mucous membranes

a. virus that causes AIDS

b. a disease that is sexually transmitted and is caused by HIV, which cripples a person's immune system

c. moist tissues that line the openings to the body

d. when two people have sex with only each other for their entire lives

e. not taking part in a particular activity

f. blood test used to test for the presence of HIV

g. condition of being infected with HIV

h. covering for the penis that helps protect both partners from sexually transmitted diseases and also helps to prevent pregnancy

Part II

Write the letter of the correct answer in the blank.

______ **9.** AIDS is

    a. survivable   c. inherited

    b. preventable   d. curable

______ **10.** HIV can infect

    a. only homosexual men

    b. only heterosexual females

    c. anyone who does certain things

    d. only people 20 years old or older

______ **11.** Which of the following is *not* true of HIV?

    a. It attacks a special kind of white blood cell, called a T4 cell.

    b. It strengthens the immune system.

    c. It can be in a person's system for years before it causes health problems.

    d. It opens the way for opportunistic infections.

______ **12.** A person with HIV

    a. can look and feel well but still infect another person

    b. may not know he or she is infected

    c. can find out if he or she has HIV through an HIV-antibody test

    d. all of the above

_______ **13.** HIV can enter the body through

     a. food   c. blood
     b. air   d. water

_______ **14.** One body fluid that can contain enough HIV to infect another person is

     a. tears   c. perspiration
     b. semen   d. urine

_______ **15.** The best way to prevent HIV infection through sexual behaviors is to

     a. delay sexual intercourse until in a monogamous relationship with a disease-free person who practices safe behaviors
     b. limit the number of partners
     c. use a latex condom
     d. avoid the use of alcohol or drugs when engaging in sex

_______ **16.** If you suspect you have been infected with HIV, you should

     a. be tested for HIV immediately and again after six months
     b. wait a few weeks for symptoms to appear
     c. tell no one as you may encounter discrimination
     d. all of the above

_______ **17.** HIV infection can be

     a. cured with nonoxynol-9   c. treated with AZT
     b. reversed with ddI   d. all of the above

_______ **18.** Medical treatment for HIV

     a. should be started before infections, as a prevention
     b. can postpone the onset of symptoms
     c. includes a vaccine to prevent the further spread of HIV infection
     d. should be obtained before having sex

_______ **19.** You can help people who are HIV-positive by

     a. feeling sorry for them
     b. treating them with respect
     c. avoiding physical contact with them
     d. encouraging them to ignore the problem

Part III . . . .

Write R on the line in front of a behavior that would put a person at risk of being infected with HIV. Write S on the line if the behavior is safe.

_______ **20.** Sharing tools for ear piercing

_______ **21.** Playing tennis

_______ **22.** Having unprotected sexual intercourse

_______ **23.** Kissing

_______ **24.** Donating blood

Part IV ·

Answer the question in the space provided.

25. Your friend confides in you that she is thinking of having sexual intercourse with her boyfriend because he is pressuring her to do so. Your friend is undecided about whether to remain abstinent or have sexual intercourse using a condom. What would you encourage your friend to do? Why? If your friend decides to have sexual intercourse, what would you tell her about condoms?

Chapter 24

Noninfectious Diseases and Disorders

Chapter Test

Part I

Match the definitions on the right with the terms on the left.

_____ **1.** atherosclerosis

_____ **2.** autoimmune disease

_____ **3.** cancer

_____ **4.** cardiovascular disease

_____ **5.** chromosome

_____ **6.** congenital disease

_____ **7.** degenerative disease

_____ **8.** gene

_____ **9.** hereditary disease

_____ **10.** noninfectious disease

a. a disease that cannot be caught from another person, animal, or organism

b. a disease caused by defective genes inherited by a child from one or both parents

c. a disease that is present from birth but is not inherited

d. structure made up of DNA

e. a short segment of DNA that is a code for a particular bit of information

f. a disease in which a person's own immune system attacks and damages an organ of his or her own body

g. narrowing of the arteries caused by a buildup of cholesterol

h. a disease that results from the gradual damage to organs over time

i. progressive damage to the heart and blood vessels

j. a disease caused by cells that have lost normal growth controls and that invade and destroy other tissues

Part II

Write the letter of the correct answer in the blank.

_____ **11.** Cataracts, heart defects, and facial deformities are three kinds of congenital diseases. Congenital diseases can be caused by

 a. over-the-counter drugs c. illegal drugs
 b. prescription drugs d. all of the above

_____ **12.** Hemophilia is a disease that is caused by the absence of a clotting factor. Therefore, after an injury, a hemophiliac bleeds not only externally but also internally. Hemophilia is a disease that is passed from a mother to her son. Hemophilia is a

 a. congenital disease c. autoimmune disease
 b. hereditary disease d. infectious disease

_____ **13.** AIDS differs from autoimmune diseases in that

 a. autoimmune diseases involve the immune system but AIDS does not
 b. AIDS is communicable but autoimmune diseases are not
 c. AIDS is triggered by a bacterium but autoimmune diseases are triggered by viruses
 d. AIDS is a degenerative disease but autoimmune diseases are not

______ **14.** Atherosclerosis can be caused by
  a. high blood cholesterol levels
  b. small injuries to the inner walls of arteries
  c. high blood pressure
  d. all of the above

______ **15.** Baby Elizabeth lies in a hospital crib. She is underweight, sickly, and has brain damage. Her mother abused cocaine while she was pregnant. The mental retardation Elizabeth suffers from is very likely due to a
  a. congenital disease   c. degenerative disease
  b. hereditary disease   d. infectious disease

______ **16.** Which of the following statements about a heart attack is *not* true?
  a. A heart attack occurs when one or more coronary arteries become blocked.
  b. Symptoms of a heart attack can include chest pain, shortness of breath, and nausea.
  c. The chances of a heart attack are lower in a person who does not smoke.
  d. If the damaged region of the heart is not too large, the heart muscle can regenerate itself.

______ **17.** Which of the following statements about cancer is *not* true?
  a. Cancer caught early is often curable.
  b. The tendency to develop some cancers may be hereditary.
  c. Getting a suntan is healthy and does not contribute to the risk of skin cancer.
  d. Tobacco products can cause cancers of the lungs, bladder, and pancreas.

Part III ·

Listed below are various types of diseases. On the line in front of each disease, write H for a hereditary disease, C for a congenital disease, A for an autoimmune disease, and D for a degenerative disease.

______ **18.** Down's syndrome

______ **19.** Multiple sclerosis

______ **20.** Fetal alcohol syndrome

______ **21.** Sickle cell anemia

______ **22.** Rheumatoid arthritis

______ **23.** Cerebral palsy

______ **24.** Osteoarthritis

Part IV . . . .

Write the answer to the question in the space provided.

25. In what ways are a heart attack and a stroke similar? In what ways are they different?

Chapter 25

Environmental and Public Health
Chapter Test

Part I ·

Match the definitions on the right with the terms on the left.

_____ **1.** conservation

_____ **2.** ecosystem

_____ **3.** environment

_____ **4.** epidemic

_____ **5.** global warming

_____ **6.** greenhouse effect

_____ **7.** nonrenewable resource

_____ **8.** pollution

_____ **9.** public health

_____ **10.** recycling

a. a system made of living things and their physical surroundings

b. trapping of heat from the sun

c. a condition that results when harmful substances contaminate the environment

d. all the nonliving things that surround and influence a living thing

e. long-term increase in the temperature of the Earth's climate

f. reusing materials

g. the wise use and protection of natural resources

h. organized efforts of a community to promote the health of its members

i. natural resource that takes millions of years to replace

j. an outbreak of a disease that affects many people in a given area

Part II ·

Write the letter of the correct answer on the line.

_____ **11.** One example of interdependency in an ecosystem is
   a. changes in seasons
   b. plants take in carbon dioxide and give off oxygen; animals take in oxygen and give off carbon dioxide
   c. water enters cracks in rocks; water freezes and breaks the rocks apart, helping to form soil
   d. weather patterns

_____ **12.** In order to have a healthy environment, there must be an adequate supply of
   a. carbon monoxide
   b. water
   c. chlorofluorocarbons
   d. coal

_____ **13.** Pollution can
   a. adversely affect the health of living things
   b. lead to cancer
   c. create shortages of water
   d. all of the above

______**14.** Which of the following is an example of responsible waste management?

    a. Use toxic products carefully.
    b. Purchase products that are sold in spray pumps instead of in aerosol cans.
    c. Recycle glass bottles.
    d. Use less electricity.

______**15.** How might you reduce water pollution?

    a. Dispose of household chemicals safely.
    b. Start a compost pile.
    c. Use high-phosphate detergents.
    d. Fix leaky faucets.

______**16.** Public health is not concerned about

    a. controlling the spread of infectious diseases
    b. developing quality health facilities
    c. immunization and antibiotic treatment
    d. regulating our gasoline supplies

______**17.** Which of the following is *not* a major public-health concern or goal in developed countries?

    a. Famine
    b. Preventive services
    c. Homelessness
    d. Teen pregnancy

______**18.** Which of the following is a local source of help for a public-health problem in your community?

    a. Department of Health and Human Services
    b. City Health Department
    c. UNESCO
    d. all of the above

______**19.** The primary health organization of the United Nations is

    a. AID
    b. UNESCO
    c. WHO
    d. ASPCA

Part III ·

Fill in each blank with the type of pollution that best completes each sentence.

20. Automobiles, factories, and power-generating plants contribute to

______________________________.

21. Cholera and gastrointestinal disorders, as well as some forms of cancer, are directly related to

______________________________.

22. An accumulation of solid waste materials that are discarded by humans adds to the problem of

________________________________.

23. Automobiles, trucks, jets, and rock concerts are sources of

________________________________.

24. Lung cancer and birth defects can be linked to ________________________________.

Part IV . . . .

Answer the question in the space provided.

25. You have just learned that your friend has been dumping used motor oil in an empty field near his house. What would you say or do to discourage him from this practice?

Being a Wise Consumer

Chapter Test

Part I

Match the terms on the left with the definitions on the right.

_____ **1.** deductible

_____ **2.** defensive medicine

_____ **3.** HMO

_____ **4.** Medicaid

_____ **5.** premium

_____ **6.** primary-care physician

_____ **7.** quackery

_____ **8.** second opinion

_____ **9.** Medicare

_____ **10.** patient's bill of rights

a. a family medicine physician

b. use of numerous diagnostic tests to avoid a lawsuit

c. an organization that offers subscribers complete medical care in return for a fixed monthly fee

d. federal aid for the elderly

e. a set fee that must be paid by an individual before health insurance begins to cover medical costs

f. a fee paid for private health insurance

g. the promotion of medical services or products that are worthless or unproven

h. basic right of human beings to get quality health care

i. the diagnosis and advice of another doctor

j. a federally financed insurance program for disabled people and low-income families

Part II

Write the letter of the correct answer in the blank.

_____ **11.** Which of the following is a source that you can use to help find a new doctor?

    a. friend   c. local hospital
    b. relative   d. all of the above

_____ **12.** One thing to know about a doctor in order to help you make a choice is

    a. how many years he or she has practiced
    b. his or her office hours
    c. his or her philosophy of treatment
    d. all of the above

_____ **13.** Which of the following is a good reason to change doctors?

    a. The doctor asks a lot of questions about your medical history.
    b. The doctor asks questions about your health habits.
    c. You observe questionable practices in the doctor's office.
    d. all of the above

_____ **14.** When talking with your doctor, you should feel
    a. you do not need to hurry
    b. reluctant to ask questions
    c. no need to ask for a second opinion
    d. all of the above

_____ **15.** It is acceptable for your doctor to
    a. hurry you if he or she has several patients waiting
    b. speak to you frankly about your health problems
    c. be upset if you suggest that you may want to seek a second opinion
    d. all of the above

_____ **16.** The Patient's Bill of Rights is
    a. your first step toward getting quality health care
    b. a legal document
    c. designed to apply only to hospital outpatient procedures
    d. all of the above

_____ **17.** Health-care costs in the United States are rising because of
    a. medical lawsuits and malpractice insurance costs
    b. defensive medicine
    c. high-tech equipment and procedures
    d. all of the above

_____ **18.** Health-care costs are a concern for many because
    a. small companies do not provide health insurance plans
    b. individuals cannot afford to pay high health insurance premiums
    c. a serious illness or injury can drain a family's savings
    d. all of the above

_____ **19.** Traditional private insurance policies
    a. do not require a premium to be paid
    b. often do not cover preventive health care
    c. pay 100 percent of medical costs
    d. all of the above

_____ **20.** Health maintenance organizations, or HMOs,
    a. require a monthly fee
    b. allow for a wide choice of physicians and hospitals
    c. are funded by the federal government
    d. all of the above

_____ **21.** State and county health departments offer services
    a. only to the poor
    b. to anyone
    c. for all health problems
    d. for preventive medicine only

_______ **22.** Your friend has told you that her mother just found out she is pregnant. Her father has been out of work for eight months. They have no health insurance and are concerned about how they will be able to pay for doctor bills. You might suggest they

    a. join an HMO
    b. contact the county health department
    c. take out a private health insurance policy
    d. call their state insurance department

_______ **23.** One should be concerned about and able to identify quackery because such claims could

    a. be a waste of one's money
    b. endanger one's health
    c. delay appropriate diagnosis and treatment
    d. all of the above

_______ **24.** One way to tell whether a product is worthless or unproven is to look for claims

    a. of a new, secret remedy
    b. of a quick cure
    c. by patients who have been cured by using the product
    d. all of the above

Part III ....

Answer the question in the space provided.

25. You have an elderly unemployed friend who is in need of medical care. What kind of health-care services would you recommend for him? Why?

____

____

____

____

____

____

____

____

____

Chapter 27

Safety and Risk Reduction

Chapter Test

Part I

Match the definitions on the right with the terms on the left.

______ **1.** accident

______ **2.** assault

______ **3.** carelessness

______ **4.** defensive driving

______ **5.** disaster

______ **6.** electrocution

______ **7.** risk

______ **8.** safety awareness

______ **9.** thunderstorm

______ **10.** tornado

a. an action that is potentially dangerous

b. inattentive behavior while performing a task

c. knowledge about risks and how to reduce them

d. an unexpected event that causes damage, injury, or death

e. expecting other motorists to do the unexpected

f. a major event that threatens the lives and safety of people in one or more communities

g. powerful short-lived storm characterized by lightning, rain, and strong winds

h. a brief storm that is characterized by wind speeds as high as 300 miles per hour

i. death resulting from electric current passing through the body

j. a personal attack in which the person is threatened or harmed

Part II

Write the letter of the correct answer in the blank.

______ **11.** The leading cause of death among people between the ages of 15 and 24 is

a. poisoning
b. falls
c. accidents
d. drowning

______ **12.** Which of the following will reduce the risk of injury in an automobile accident?

a. Not riding with someone who has been drinking or using drugs
b. Driving defensively
c. Always wearing your seat belt
d. All of the above

______ **13.** Which of the following is not a contributing factor in motor-vehicle accidents?

a. Expecting other drivers to do the unexpected
b. Letting someone who has been drinking drive home
c. Failing to stop at a stop sign
d. Turning left without signaling

_______ **14.** Greg's 19-year-old brother, Rob, just brought home a used motorcycle. Rob wants to give Greg a ride on the bike. Greg isn't sure he wants to go. What question does Greg need answered before he makes a decision?

    a. How much experience does Rob have riding a motorcycle?
    b. Is there a helmet that he can wear?
    c. Is he properly dressed?
    d. All of the above

_______ **15.** When riding a bicycle, it is important to

    a. stay on the sidewalk
    b. ride against the flow of traffic
    c. use hand signals to change direction and speed
    d. all of the above

_______ **16.** Which of the following can lead to a bicycle accident?

    a. Not wearing a helmet
    b. A chain that is well greased
    c. Riding through water-filled holes
    d. A properly inflated tire

_______ **17.** Almost 82 percent of accidents in the workplace are due to

    a. disregarding safety requirements
    b. using faulty equipment
    c. working with toxic chemicals
    d. working in unsafe conditions

_______ **18.** Jason wants to play hockey. First he must learn how to skate. He has had several lessons and is now practicing skating fast and turning quickly. Perhaps the most important piece of equipment Jason should wear during practice to reduce his risk of a serious injury is

    a. elbow pads   c. shinguards
    b. kneepads   d. a helmet

Part III ·

Listed below are several ways to reduce the potential for injury. On the line in front of each statement, write the hazard that is reduced.

________________ **19.** Sprinkle salt on icy sidewalks and stairs.

________________ **20.** Keep rags, paper, and other combustible materials away from the furnace.

________________ **21.** Do not go near any wires that are on the ground.

________________ **22.** Keep gasoline for lawn mowers in specially made and marked gasoline cans.

________________ **23.** Always swim where there is a lifeguard.

________________ **24.** Stay away from windows to avoid getting cut by broken glass.

Part IV . . . .

Answer the question in the space provided.

25. In terms of personal behavior and what an individual can control, what is the difference between accidents that occur in the home and natural disasters? How can you eliminate or minimize the risk of each?

First Aid and CPR

Chapter Test

Part I ....

Match the terms on the left with the definitions on the right.

_____ **1.** cardiopulmonary resuscitation

_____ **2.** heat exhaustion

_____ **3.** heatstroke

_____ **4.** Heimlich maneuver

_____ **5.** hypothermia

_____ **6.** shock

a. a condition in which the body's vital processes are severely depressed

b. series of sharp thrusts to the abdomen, used to dislodge an object from the airway

c. a condition caused by the loss of water and salt

d. a loss of body heat that causes the body temperature to fall well below normal

e. a lifesaving procedure designed to revive a victim who is not breathing

f. a life-threatening emergency caused by prolonged exposure to heat

Part II ....

Write the letter of the correct answer in the blank.

_____ **7.** Lionel's brother cuts his finger on a saw blade. The cut is deep and bleeding badly. What is the first thing Lionel should do?

     a. Wash the cut with clean water.
     b. Cover the cut with a clean dressing and apply pressure.
     c. Raise the cut above the level of his brother's heart.
     d. Call for help.

_____ **8.** Sara is baby-sitting for her neighbor's children. The 5-year-old child suddenly collapses, unconscious. Sara sends the 8-year-old to call for help. What should Sara do next?
     a. Check for a pulse.
     b. Administer CPR.
     c. Tilt the child's head back to open the airway.
     d. Check to see if the child is breathing.

_____ **9.** It is a hot, humid summer day. Jason had just finished jogging 10 miles when he stopped by your house to play basketball. After playing for about 20 minutes, Jason says he does not feel well. He feels nauseated and dizzy. His skin is clammy. You have him lie down in the shade. What is the next thing you should do?
     a. Treat for shock.
     b. Do nothing, but observe him carefully.
     c. Give him water to drink.
     d. Take him to a hospital emergency room.

______ **10.** If you are the first person to arrive on the scene of a medical emergency, you should

    a. survey the scene for possible danger to you or the victim
    b. rescue the person whose life is endangered
    c. send for medical help
    d. all of the above

______ **11.** You and several friends are playing football. One of your friends gets tackled hard; you hear a sharp, cracking noise. Your friend yells out and grabs his arm. Everyone stops playing. Another friend leaves to get help. What should you do next?

    a. Try to straighten out your friend's arm.
    b. Treat for shock.
    c. Build a splint to immobilize the arm.
    d. Provide padding around the suspected broken arm.

______ **12.** You are watching your friend, Ann, ride her horse over a series of jumps. Going over one fence, she falls. She doesn't get up, so you run over to her. She complains that her neck and right wrist hurt. You send someone for help. What is the next thing you should do?

    a. Place your hands on either side of her head to keep it still.
    b. Remove her riding helmet.
    c. Treat her wrist for fracture.
    d. Help her sit up so you can better assess her condition.

______ **13.** Terrence is visiting his grandmother. He is helping her prepare lunch when she begins to experience chest pain, weakness, and a weak and irregular pulse. She is still conscious and able to talk. Terrence knows his grandmother has a heart condition. What should he do first?

    a. Administer CPR.
    b. Have his grandmother sit or lie down, propping up her head.
    c. Call for help.
    d. Help give her any heart medication she needs to take.

______ **14.** Alice is in a restaurant. She notices a young man falling off his chair and onto the floor. He is unconscious. When Alice gets to him, he starts having convulsions. What should Alice do?

    a. Administer the Heimlich maneuver.
    b. Try to restrain him.
    c. Pry open his mouth and use a spoon to hold his tongue down.
    d. Loosen tight clothing and remove large objects from the area surrounding him so he won't harm himself.

______ **15.** Carlos gets caught in an early snowstorm. The temperature drops quickly. His car gets stuck in the snow three blocks from home. Wearing a light jacket, Carlos walks home. When he gets there, he is shivering. What should Carlos do first?

    a. Run his hands under warm water.
    b. Wrap himself in blankets.
    c. Take a warm shower.
    d. Fix himself a glass of hot chocolate.

_______ **16.** Jessica is four years old. She begins crying and tells you her stomach hurts, her throat burns, and she feels like vomiting. You notice a strange odor on her breath and an empty bottle next to her. What should you do first?

- a. Call the poison control center.
- b. Give Jessica syrup of ipecac to make her vomit.
- c. Treat for shock.
- d. Try to find out what Jessica may have swallowed by asking her.

Part III

Complete the chart below.

EMERGENCIES			
Event	Assessment	Possible cause or injury	First aid
A man clutches his chest and falls, unconscious, to the ground.	There is no breathing or pulse.	**17.**	**18.**
You pick up a hot pan.	Skin is red but no blisters are forming.	**19.**	**20.**
A person in a restaurant suddenly stands up and grabs his or her throat.	**21.**	choking	**22.**
A child is running and falls. The child grabs his or her ankle.	**23.**	sprain	**24.**

Part IV

Answer the question in the space provided.

25. What can you do to protect yourself from health emergencies related to hot weather?

____

____

____

____

____

____

Chapter 1

Health and Wellness: A Quality of Life
Alternative Assessment

Read the following paragraph, and then answer the questions below:

Pete and Tanya are teenagers. When he comes home from school, Pete prefers to watch television and snack on soda and potato chips. If his parents are not home, Pete sometimes sneaks liquor from the liquor cabinet and adds it to his soda. Pete has also begun smoking with his friends. Tanya, on the other hand, prefers to ride her bicycle for several miles when she gets home from school. She does not, however, wear a helmet. Tanya also enjoys soda and potato chips, but she tries to include fresh fruits and vegetables in her diet. Tanya often stays up very late, making it difficult for her to get up in the morning. As a result, she has to hurry to get to school on time, often skips breakfast, and is tired and very hungry by the end of her second class.

1. Wellness can be considered as part of a continuum—from illness and risk of early death to wellness and likelihood of long life. Draw a line that would illustrate a wellness continuum. Label one end "Illness" and the other end "Wellness." Label the middle of your line "Neither ill nor well."

2. Indicate where Pete would fall on your wellness continuum.

3. Indicate where Tanya would fall on your wellness continuum.

4. What behaviors would move Pete and Tanya closer to wellness?

____

____

____

5. Where do you think you fall on the wellness continuum?

____

6. List four behaviors you could practice that would help you move closer to wellness, longer life, and a higher quality of life.

____

____

____

____

NAME ___________ CLASS ___________ DATE ___________

Making Responsible Decisions
Alternative Assessment

1. In the spaces below, write a story in which a student encounters a dangerous or high-pressure situation that forces him or her to make a very difficult decision. Describe how the student feels. Do not finish the story.

____

____

____

____

____

____

____

____

____

____

____

2. Trade papers with a partner, and complete his or her story in the space below, having the character use the decision-making model to handle the difficult situation.

____

____

____

____

____

____

____

____

____

____

____

____

____

____

Chapter 3

Physical Fitness

Alternative Assessment

Answer each of the sentences in the spaces provided.

1. How can exercise benefit a person mentally and physically?

2. Which of the fitness categories would concern you most if you wanted to become a marathon runner? a piano mover? a ballet dancer?

3. How do aerobic exercises benefit your heart?

4. When doing anaerobic exercises, what three things do you need to be concerned about to improve your overall physical fitness?

5. How are steroids dangerous?

6. If you wanted to improve your circulatory and respiratory systems, what exercises could you choose?

7. In a weight-control program, how is exercise beneficial?

8. Why is sleep an important part of physical fitness?

NAME   CLASS   DATE

Alternative Assessment

Use what you have learned about nutrition to complete the following exercise.

Your friend Gavin has asked you to help him modify his eating habits. He has given you a menu of what he commonly eats in one day. Review the menu and evaluate it by answering the questions that follow.

Gavin's Menu

Breakfast	sweet roll, soda
Lunch	one slice of cheese pizza
Snack	chocolate bar
Dinner	pork chops, green beans, two helpings of mashed potatoes, apple sauce, two rolls, two pieces of cherry pie
Snack	milk, two chocolate-chip cookies

1. Evaluate Gavin's diet. Is he getting too much or too little of any food groups?

____

____

____

____

____

____

2. If you could revise Gavin's diet, what items would you replace? What would you replace them with?

____

____

____

____

____

____

Weight Management and Eating Disorders
Alternative Assessment

**Eating disorders, such as anorexia nervosa and bulimia, can seriously affect
one's health. Both disorders can lead to malnutrition. Read the following story,
and then answer the questions that follow.**

Your best friend, Christine, has been taking ballet lessons since she was three years old. She
wants to be a professional dancer. Her parents want the same for her and are constantly
pushing her to practice and to try out for various programs. Christine is always concerned about
her weight as well as her body image. She is very conscious about what and how much she
eats. You tell her she looks terrific and is not at all overweight. In fact, you think she may be
underweight. But Christine disagrees with you. She confides in you that her dance instructor told
her she was too fat. Her dance instructor makes all the girls in the dance class weigh in before
every lesson. If any girl weighs too much, the instructor makes her sit in front of a mirror during
the entire lesson. Christine told you she had to do this once and it was so humiliating that now
she'll often make herself vomit before a lesson so she won't weigh too much.

1. What concerns would you have about Christine?

____

____

____

____

2. You talk to Christine about these concerns, but she tells you there is nothing to worry about. Would you
talk to Christine's parents about your concerns? Why or why not? If you did, what would you say?

____

____

____

____

____

3. Besides talking to Christine's parents, what other things could you do to help her?

____

____

____

____

Alternative Assessment

It is important to brush your teeth twice daily and to floss them once a day. To find out how well you brush and floss, follow the steps below.

Step 1 Obtain disclosing tablets from your dentist or local chapter of the American Dental Association. Chew one disclosing tablet until it is dissolved and then swish it around in your mouth. Spit out the dissolved disclosing tablet in a sink.

Step 2 Observe your teeth in a mirror. The dye in the disclosing tablet stains any plaque that is present on your teeth.

Step 3 Use the scale on the right as a guide to monitor how much plaque is present in your mouth.

▶ **1.** At what level would you rate the plaque on your teeth? _______

Step 4 Floss and brush your teeth as outlined in your text.

Step 5 Chew another disclosing tablet as described in Step 1.

Step 6 Look at your teeth in a mirror again. Use the scale in Step 3 to evaluate the amount of plaque on your teeth.

▶ **2.** At what level would you rate the plaque on your teeth after brushing and flossing? _______

▶ **3.** How effective were your flossing and brushing techniques?

____

▶ **4.** How might you improve your flossing and brushing techniques?

____

▶ **5.** Why is it important to remove as much plaque as possible from your teeth every day?

____

▶ **6.** Why is it important to see your dentist regularly?

____

____

____

LEVEL	AMOUNT AND AREAS OF PLAQUE
0	No plaque present
1	Small amount of stain between teeth
2	Stain between teeth and a thin line of stain along the gum line
3	Stain between the teeth, along gum line, and covering about $\frac{1}{3}$ of one or more teeth
4	Stain between the teeth, along gum line, and covering about $\frac{2}{3}$ of one or more teeth
5	Stain between the teeth, along gum line, and covering entire surface of several teeth

Chapter 7

Mental and Emotional Health
Alternative Assessment

Part I . . . .

Below are four things you can do to promote your mental health. What are 10 more things you can do?

1. Express your feelings to others.

2. Try to do your best without expecting to be perfect.

3. Keep disappointments in perspective.

4. Avoid using alcohol and drugs.

5. ____

6. ____

7. ____

8. ____

9. ____

10. ____

11. ____

12. ____

13. ____

14. ____

Part II . . . .

Answer the question on the lines provided.

15. If you feel you are having problems controlling a particular emotion, why should you seek the help of a mental-health professional?

____

____

____

____

____

Building Self-Esteem

Alternative Assessment

Part I ....

The first step in raising your self-esteem is to accept yourself as a unique and special person. In the following exercise, design your own coat of arms to serve as a reminder of your personal strengths and goals.

Questions About Your Self-Esteem

1. What is your greatest achievement? Draw a symbol of your achievement in section A of the drawing entitled "Coat of Arms."

2. What are three things that you are good at? Illustrate your answer in section B of the coat of arms.

3. What is one challenge you would like to take on? Illustrate your answer in section C of the coat of arms.

4. What is a group, group activity, or volunteer organization you belong to or would like to join? Illustrate your answer in section D of the coat of arms.

5. What is one thing about yourself that you are trying to improve? Illustrate your answer in section E of the coat of arms.

Coat of Arms

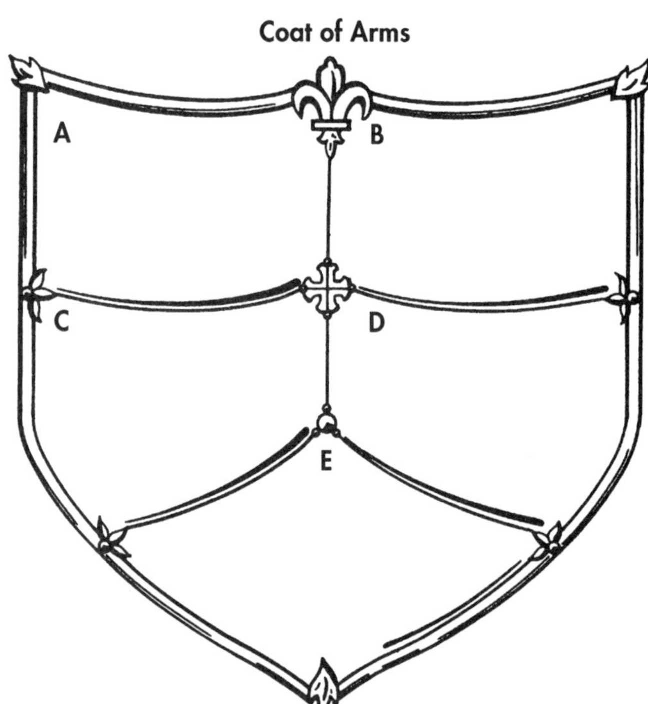

Part II ....

Answer the questions in the spaces provided.

6. How might your answers to "Questions About Your Self-Esteem" be a reflection of the influence that others could have on you?

____

____

____

7. What kinds of things could you do to raise your self-esteem?

____

____

____

Managing Stress

Alternative Assessment

Part I

In the space below, draw a rough sketch of yourself. Considering what you have learned from this chapter, write down the names of illnesses that can arise from stress and connect them with a line to the part of the body that is affected.

Part II

1. In the space below, use the stress model to write a story in which a student encounters a stressful situation. Describe how the student feels, including at least five of the common symptoms of stress. Do not finish the story.

    ____

    ____

    ____

    ____

    ____

    ____

    ____

    ____

2. Trade papers with a partner, and complete his or her story on a separate piece of paper, having the character use selective awareness to handle the stressful situation.

Chapter 10

Alternative Assessment

Part I •

Form groups of six students. Copy each of the three situations below on a piece of paper. Fold each paper in half and place it in a container.

- A 4-year-old asks his or her parent several questions about death after seeing a dead animal.
- An elderly grandparent talks with his or her teenage grandchild about coping with the recent divorce of the child's parents.
- A teenager goes to a funeral home to pay condolences to a classmate whose parent died unexpectedly.

Part II •

Members of each group should now divide into pairs. One person from each pair should draw a situation from the container. Each pair should role-play the situation that was chosen, allowing other members of the group to comment on the role-play afterward.

Part III •

Answer these questions in the spaces provided.

1. Recall childhood experiences with death.
   a. What are your earliest memories concerning death?

   ____

   b. How was death explained to you?

   ____

2. Would you explain death to a 4-year-old differently than to a teenager? Why or why not?

   ____

3. In the role-playing of the grandparent and the grandchild, at what stage of acceptance was the grandchild? How do you know?

   ____

4. As a child, were you allowed to attend the funeral of a family member or friend? If not, why? If you attended a funeral, how did you feel?

   ____

5. What is the most important thing you have learned in this chapter about loss?

   ____

6. What is the most important thing you have learned in this chapter about grieving?

   ____

Chapter 11

Alternative Assessment

Suicide is a serious problem. It is one of the leading causes of death among teenagers. Suicide can affect all kinds of people—young, old, rich, poor, female, male. Suicides can often be prevented if people recognize the warning signs and know how to help a person considering suicide.

Below are the roles for this exercise:

    a. person considering suicide
    b. boyfriend or girlfriend of the person considering suicide
    c. another friend of the person considering suicide
    d. school counselor
    e. parent

1. Form into groups of five. Have each person in a group write the description of one role on a small piece of paper. The description should include the way the person will respond to the situation—whether that response is helpful or not. The role of the person considering suicide should be described as a depressed, troubled teenager. Fold each description in half, and place the folded papers into a container.

2. Each student in the group must draw one of the papers from the container and play the role of the person described.

3. The student playing the role of the person considering suicide should begin the role-playing. The others should respond as directed in their descriptions. After the role-playing is complete, the suicidal person should tell how the responses of the others made him or her feel. If the outcome was not good, the group could replay the scene giving more helpful responses.

4. Summarize your group's responses in the space below.

____

____

____

____

____

____

____

____

Chapter 12

The Use, Misuse, and Abuse of Drugs

Alternative Assessment

Choose one of the following topics:

a. the use, misuse, and abuse of drugs

b. the three types of OTC drugs and their uses

c. the effects of common drug types

d. appropriate use of medicines

Prepare a multimedia presentation to inform an audience of your peers about one of these topics. In other words, use more than one medium, such as a slide show and a recorded message, to get your message across. Be as creative as possible. Summarize your presentation in the lines below.

Alcohol: A Dangerous Drug
Alternative Assessment

Think about the various advertisements that you have seen and how the media portrays the use of alcohol.

Answer the questions in the spaces provided.

1. Describe an advertisement for alcohol you have seen in which alcohol use appeared glamorous or fun.

2. Give five examples of short-term or long-term effects of alcohol use and abuse that are not glamorous or fun.

3. What types of behavior would be considered responsible in terms of consuming alcohol?

4. In what ways could the media promote responsible behavior concerning alcohol use?

Tobacco: Hazardous and Addictive

Alternative Assessment

The dangers of tobacco use are well known and well documented. Because so many people are aware of these risks, today fewer people than ever use tobacco. However, many people still ignore the warnings and use tobacco products. Use the knowledge you have gained from this chapter to answer the questions below.

1. Why would a city consider passing a law that would ban smoking in all public places? Would you support such a law? Explain your answer.

____

____

____

2. A friend of yours lights up a cigarette while riding in the car with you and your younger sister. When you ask her to put the cigarette out, she says, "Why? All of that stuff about second-hand smoke is silly. I'll bet the air outside the car is just as bad." How would you respond?

____

____

____

3. Your friend Richard has decided to quit smoking. He has decided to chew tobacco instead. He says that it will satisfy his craving for nicotine without harming his health. What information could you give Richard that would prove otherwise?

____

____

____

4. In the space below, list five harmful chemicals found in cigarettes. Beside each chemical, draw a picture to illustrate either how the chemical affects the body or how else the chemical has been used.

Chapter 15

Other Drugs of Abuse

Alternative Assessment

Part I ·

Read the paragraph below, and answer the questions that follow.

Imagine that Diana, a friend of yours, has started taking amphetamines. When you ask her why she takes them, she says, "They give me so much energy. I don't have to sleep, I'm more fun to be around, and it feels like I never have to eat! My life is easier *and* I'm losing weight!"

1. What symptoms is Diana experiencing when she takes amphetamines?

____

____

2. What is happening to Diana's body to make her experience these symptoms?

____

____

____

3. What health problems could Diana experience if she does not stop taking amphetamines?

____

____

4. What negative social and academic consequences could Diana experience if she becomes addicted to amphetamines?

____

____

5. Based on what you know about exercise, nutrition, and stress management, what are some healthful activities that Diana could do to feel more energetic without taking amphetamines?

____

____

____

Part II ·

On a separate sheet of paper, make up your own scenario in which a peer is taking a drug. Include the way the drug makes them feel and their reasons for taking the drugs. When you are finished, write down a few questions that evaluate the negative consequences of drug use. Have a partner read your paragraph and answer the questions that follow it.

Chapter 16

Reproduction and the Early Years of Life
Alternative Assessment

Answer the following questions:

1. Why is it important for a person to know about his or her own reproductive system?

2. Why is it important for a person to know about the reproductive system of the opposite sex?

3. Imagine that you are a parent and your child comes to you and asks, "Where was I before I was born?" How would you answer this question? Give reasons for why you would answer this way.

Chapter 17

Adolescence: Relationships and Responsibilities
Alternative Assessment

Read the paragraph and follow the directions below.

Jill is confused. She and her boyfriend, Todd, have been dating for six months. Lately Todd has been asking her to have sexual intercourse. So far, Jill has told Todd that she wants to wait until she is married to have sex. Her parents have always told her that she should wait, and she knows that they would be disappointed if they found out that she had sex before marriage. Even though she is attracted to Todd and cares about him, Jill feels that she could easily wait. But Todd says he really needs to have sex. He says that he is at his sexual peak and that it is torture for him to wait. Jill is afraid that Todd will eventually feel rejected and seek another relationship if she keeps refusing him. Plus, Todd has said that Jill's parents have forced their morals on her, and that if she learned to make up her own mind, she would not be so resistant.

1. What are Jill's concerns and priorities? Explain how you feel about each of these concerns and priorities.

____

____

____

2. What are Todd's concerns and priorities? Explain how you feel about each of these concerns and priorities.

____

____

____

3. Explain why not knowing how you feel about sexual intercourse is a good reason not to practice it.

____

____

____

4. Todd makes it sound like having sexual intercourse is an act of independence. Explain how having intercourse with Todd would show Jill's dependence and not her independence.

____

____

____

5. Jill does not feel comfortable about having intercourse. How would Todd be showing respect for Jill by not pressuring her to do what makes her uncomfortable?

____

____

____

6. How could Jill use one or more of the communication methods described in this chapter to help Todd understand that she wants to wait? What could Todd do to be a good listener?

____

____

____

____

7. Why would it be a good idea for Jill to talk with Todd at a time when they are not being physically intimate?

____

____

____

____

8. What could Todd do or whom could he talk to to handle his emotions?

____

____

____

____

9. Suppose that Jill decided to have intercourse with Todd and then realized that it was a mistake. How could Jill tell Todd that she does not want to have sex again?

____

____

____

____

NAME ______________ CLASS ______ DATE ______

Chapter 18

Adulthood, Marriage, and Parenthood

Alternative Assessment

Part I

Andrea is 17 years old and a junior in high school. Her boyfriend, Paul, is 20 and a freshman at the community college. Both have part-time jobs. They have been dating for eight months. They have decided that they want to get married in the summer after Andrea's 18th birthday.

Use the chart below to list some pros and cons about this marriage.

PROS	CONS

Part II

Answer the questions in the spaces provided.

1. Based on the pros and cons, would you advise Andrea and Paul to get married at the end of the school year or to wait? Explain.

____

____

2. In a successful marriage, spouses share responsibilities. What do you think should be your responsibilities in a marriage?

____

____

3. What responsibilities do you think should be your spouse's?

____

____

4. How would you go about solving a conflict about how the responsibilities should be shared?

____

____

Chapter 19

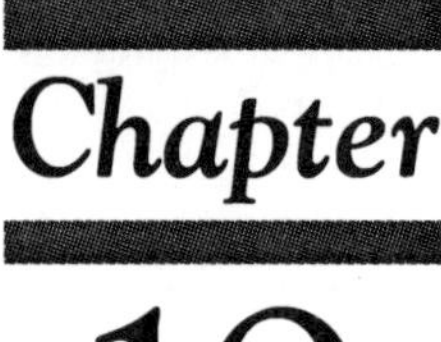

Alternative Assessment

Dysfunctional families experience high levels of stress, which can lead to personal illness, the breakdown of relationships, and family violence. Although it is impossible to eliminate all family stress, it is possible to reduce it. Knowing and understanding the characteristics and functions of a healthy family is the first step in reducing family stress.

Read the statements below.

A. There are many things this family just doesn't talk about.

B. Tempers do not flare easily in this family.

C. Disagreements happen, but usually everyone is willing to compromise.

D. This family does not adjust well when problems or big changes take place.

E. It seems that some family members listen but don't really hear what other members are saying.

F. The members of this family usually try hard to understand one another.

G. The members of this family express their love and respect for each other.

H. When it comes to family leisure time, this family sometimes finds it is hard to decide on something that all family members want to do.

Answer the questions in the spaces provided using the statements above. Write the letters of the statements on the line.

1. Which statements reflect normal characteristics of a healthy family?

____

2. Which statements may reflect unhealthy family characteristics?

____

3. Read each statement again. What changes, if any, would you make to each statement to reflect how you would like your family to be when you have children?

____

____

____

____

____

____

Chapter 20

Preventing Abuse and Violence

Alternative Assessment

Read the paragraph below, and answer the questions that follow.

Kathy is 11 years old. Her father, a single parent, works hard to pay the rent each month. Because Kathy's father spends many of his evenings "unwinding" at a local bar, Kathy and her three-year-old brother, Colin, often spend their evenings alone. Kathy manages to get along pretty well. She does the laundry and keeps the house clean. For dinner she and Colin usually eat cereal. When her father has gone to the store, sometimes she fixes hot dogs. Kathy's father pays for a baby-sitter to take care of Colin while Kathy is at school, but the baby-sitter often yells at Colin for no apparent reason. Kathy has even seen the baby-sitter hit her brother on the back. It wasn't a hard blow, but it upset Colin. Lately Kathy has been worried about Colin's health. He has had a bad ear infection for several days now, and their father has not taken Colin to the doctor. Last night Colin wouldn't stop crying. Kathy's father threatened to hit Colin, and then left the house. Kathy's father has threatened to hit them many times, but he has never so much as slapped either of them. Kathy is glad that her father is not abusive.

1. What forms of abuse are illustrated in the scenario above?

____

____

2. How could Kathy's father be considered abusive, even though he hasn't hit his children? Explain your answer.

____

____

____

3. What could Kathy do to get help for herself and her brother?

____

____

____

4. What behaviors could Kathy's father change to take better care of his children? Explain your answer.

____

____

____

Chapter 21

Infectious Diseases

Alternative Assessment

Read the paragraph below, and answer the questions that follow.

Ethan has been ill for several days. He's been miserable with a fever, muscle aches, coughing, and exhaustion. He has also had pain in his sinuses. Ethan wonders what disease he has and who gave it to him. He thinks he has narrowed it down to four people. Frank, a boy in Ethan's gym class, has tuberculosis. Frank has known about his disease for several years and takes precautions not to spread it. But Ethan thinks he may have caught the disease from Frank during a basketball game. Another classmate, Rhonda, has been out sick for about two weeks with mononucleosis. Rhonda sits next to Ethan in Biology, but they have never spoken. Ethan's best friend, Chris, came to school last week with aching muscles, a cough, and a fever. Chris and Ethan ate lunch together just before Chris was sent home from school, but Ethan was careful not to share food or beverages. Some of Chris' symptoms are like Ethan's, but Chris did not have sinus pain, and he was sick over a week ago. Ethan's younger brother Daniel got sick with chickenpox at the same time as Ethan. Daniel is the same age that Ethan was when Ethan had chickenpox.

1. Of the four people described in the story, which would you rule out as having carried the agent of Ethan's disease? Explain your answer.

____

____

____

____

2. What should Ethan do to find out what is really causing his illness?

____

____

____

____

3. What steps should Ethan take to prevent the spreading of his illness?

____

____

____

____

Chapter 22

Alternative Assessment

Part I

There are no vaccines to prevent sexually transmitted diseases. And there is no such thing as "completely safe sex." However, some at-risk behaviors are more dangerous than others. For each of the behaviors listed below, evaluate the risk of transmitting an STD. Include, if you can, how the behavior could transmit an STD and which STDs could be transmitted.

1. Hugging:

2. Open-mouth kissing:

3. Oral sex:

4. Vaginal intercourse with proper use of a latex condom with and without spermicide:

Alternative Assessment

Many people who know that they have been exposed to HIV do not get tested because they are afraid of getting bad results. These people sometimes use unrealistic explanations to convince themselves that they are not at risk. Consider the following scenario.

Cassandra and a few of her friends decided to pierce their ears using a sewing needle and an ice cube. The needle was wiped off with tissue after each use. Cassandra later found out that one of her friends is HIV positive. She has drawn a flowchart to help her decide what to do.

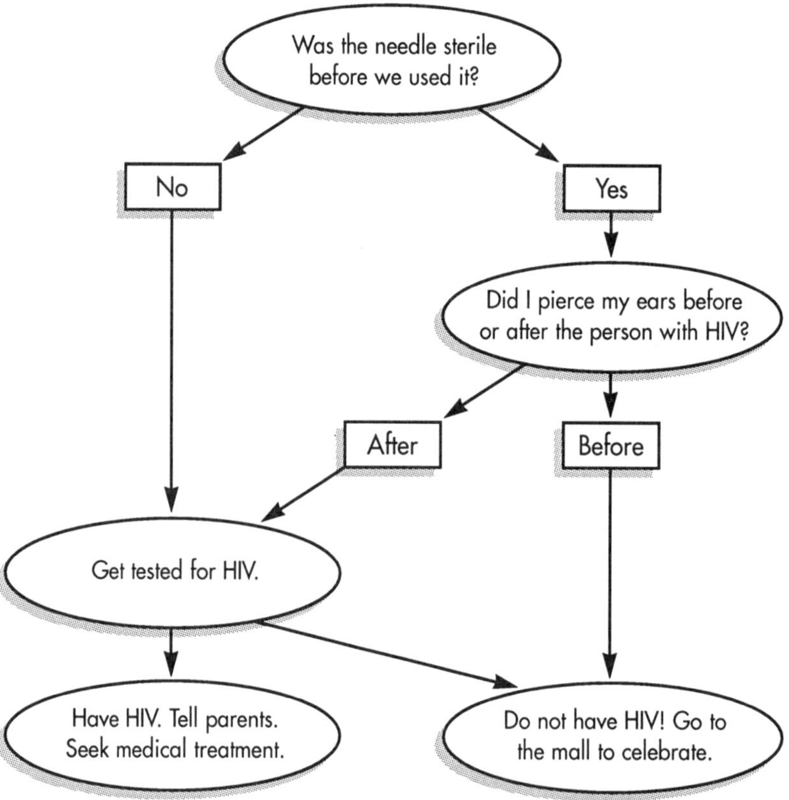

Although Cassandra has carefully analyzed her situation, there are some serious flaws in her logic. What parts of the flowchart shows decisions that put Cassandra's health at risk? What do you think Cassandra should do in this situation?

____

____

____

____

____

Chapter 24

Noninfectious Diseases and Disorders

Alternative Assessment

Study the pie charts below, and then answer the questions that follow.

1997 Cancer Incidence by Site and Sex			
Male		**Female**	
Prostate	334500	Breast	180200
Lung	98300	Lung	79800
Colon & Rectum	66400	Colon & Rectum	64800
Urinary bladder	39500	Uterus	34900
Non-Hodgkin's lymphoma	30300	Ovary	26800
Melanoma of the skin	22900	Non-Hodgkin's lymphoma	23300
Oral cavity	20900	Melanoma of the skin	17400
Kidney	17100	Urinary bladder	15000
Leukemia	15900	Cervix	14500
Stomach	14000	Pancreas	14200
All other	126000	All other	125700

1997 Cancer Deaths by Site and Sex			
Male		**Female**	
Lung	94400	Lung	66000
Prostate	41800	Breast	43900
Colon & Rectum	27000	Colon & Rectum	27900
Pancreas	13500	Pancreas	14600
Non-Hodgkin's lymphoma	12400	Ovary	14200
Leukemia	11770	Non-Hodgkin's lymphoma	11400
Esophagus	8700	Leukemia	9540
Stomach	8300	Uterus	6000
Urinary bladder	7800	Brain	6000
Liver	7500	Stomach	5700
All other	60930	All other	60660

American Cancer Society: Adapted from "Leading Sites of New Cancer Cases and Deaths -- 1997 Estimates" from *American Cancer Society Website*. Copyright © 1997 by American Cancer Society, Inc. Available Online at http://www.cancer.org/97tabp9.html

1. What are the three most common types of cancer found in women? in men? Which three types of cancer cause the most deaths in women? in men?

2. What one lifestyle change could greatly reduce a person's chance of developing lung cancer?

3. What are the seven warning signs of cancer?

4. Why is it important to know these warning signs and to act upon any of these signs if they appear?

5. What are three things you can do to reduce your risk of developing cancer?

Chapter 25

Alternative Assessment

Part I

Pollution harms the physical environment and all the living things in the environment. When pollution is not controlled, the air you breathe, the water you drink, the land you use, and even the food you eat become contaminated and unhealthy.

1. Form a group with three other students.

2. Each person should have a 4 x 6 in. index card. One person should write at the top of his or her card "Water Pollution." A second person should write "Air Pollution." A third person should write "Land Pollution" and the fourth "Noise Pollution."

3. They should also write the following headings on each card: "Cause," "Ways to Reduce Pollution," and "Benefits of Reducing Pollution."

4. Everyone should write one cause of the type of pollution that is listed at the top of his or her card, one way to reduce this type of pollution, and one benefit of reducing this type of pollution.

5. Now, everyone should pass his or her card to the person on the right.

6. After everyone passes his or her card, repeat Steps 4 and 5 three more times. No one should repeat a statement that already appears on the card.

7. When everyone has his or her original card, the cards should be placed face up on a table. As a group, examine and discuss the statements written on the cards.

Part II

Answer the questions in the spaces provided.

1. What could each of you do as an individual to reduce each type of pollution?

2. What could you do as a group to reduce each type of pollution?

3. Why do you think it is important for people to understand the benefits of reducing pollution?

Being a Wise Consumer

Alternative Assessment

Get Into Good Health . . .

Do you want to stay healthy? Treat yourself <u>Before</u> you get sick . . . with **NaturHerb.**

NaturHerb was created by Mother Nature herself to prevent illnesses of <u>all</u> kinds.

Share the secrets of the Orient, and live longer!!!

When your child is ill, look to **ComfortTabs**

The American Medical Association together with the American Academy of Pediatrics has recently endorsed **ComfortTabs** for the treatment of cold symptoms in children.

Aspirin-free, nonirritating **ComfortTabs** soothes the child and lets nature take its healing course.

Vitamin C May Prevent Cancer

Recent studies have shown that a vitamin you already take every day plays a role in preventing cancer.

Longevity Formula-C is superior to ordinary vitamin C in several ways. It is absorbed more quickly and thoroughly into the body, and it has more staying power.

Try Longevity Formula-C!

Study these three advertisements. Then answer the following questions:

1. Which advertisement is the least believable? Explain.

2. Which advertisement is probably the most accurate? Explain your answer.

3. Which advertisement would you want to find out more about? Why?

4. What types of questions might you ask about the advertisement you identified in question 3?

5. Could you use your primary care physician as a source to ask questions about these advertisements and their claims? Explain.

Safety and Risk Reduction

Alternative Assessment

Part I ·

Read the paragraph below, and then fill in the chart that follows.

There had been a constant, heavy rain for over twelve hours. Mario was driving home from work when he heard the news bulletin about the possibility of a flash flood. As he approached the bridge that crossed a small river, everyone was slowing down. Mario could see that the river had risen above the pavement and that the water was flowing swiftly. Mario watched one car after another slowly drive through the water that covered the pavement. He also watched other cars turn around instead of attempting to cross the bridge. He wasn't sure what to do. If he turned around and took another route home, it could take him 45 minutes to get there. If he crossed the bridge, he could be home in 20 minutes.

1. Advantages of crossing bridge	**2.** Risks of crossing bridge	**3.** Advantages of turning around	**4.** Risks of turning around

Part II ·

Review the completed chart above, and then answer the questions below in the spaces provided.

5. Should Mario cross the bridge or not? Explain.

____

____

____

____

6. How might using common sense and decision-making skills prevent an accident?

____

____

____

____

Chapter 28

First Aid and CPR

Alternative Assessment

Part I . . . .

Any substance that is swallowed, breathed in, injected, or absorbed by the body and that interferes with the body's normal function is a poison. Some poisons are familiar, such as cleaning chemicals, animal poisons, and pesticides. However, many common household substances can be poisonous. For example, aspirin is a useful medication and is ordinarily safe. Yet each year more children die of aspirin overdoses than from any other familiar poison.

Most poisoning can be prevented if one is aware of poisons in and around the home. Small children are at a higher risk for poisoning. That is because they are curious and often put whatever they find into their mouth. Also, it doesn't take a large amount of a substance to interfere with a child's normal body functions.

In the space below, list at least ten substances in your home that could be poisonous.

____

____

____

____

____

____

Part II . . . .

List five things you can do to prevent or prepare for an accidental poisoning in your home.

1. ____

____

2. ____

____

3. ____

____

4. ____

____

5. ____

____

Answer Key

Chapter Tests

Chapter 1

Part I
1. d
2. f
3. e
4. j
5. a
6. c
7. b
8. i
9. g
10. h

Part II
11. Illness
12. Emotional Growth
13. Optimal Health or Wellness
14. Death
15. Average Health

Part III
16. d
17. d
18. d
19. c
20. b
21. a
22. d
23. c

Part IV
24. Answers will vary. Students might answer that Rob is putting his total health at risk. Smoking cigarettes and marijuana, drinking alcohol, and taking the risk of contracting a sexually transmitted disease affect his physical health. Smoking marijuana and drinking alcohol can affect his mental, emotional, and social health, too. Although Rob feels fine, these behaviors will eventually cause health problems. The drinking and use of drugs could lead to a long term physical ailment or an accident that could cost Rob his life.
25. Answers might include avoiding smoking and drinking alcohol or taking drugs, avoiding risky sexual behavior, exercising regularly, talking with a trusted friend or family member about concerns, and doing things that will lead to positive self-esteem. Accept any answers that will move the student toward wellness.

Chapter 2

Part I
1. c
2. d
3. b
4. e
5. f
6. a

Part II
7. c
8. b
9. d
10. b
11. a
12. c
13. d
14. c
15. b
16. d

Part III
17. S, L
18. S, L
19. S, L
20. S, L
21. L
22. L

Part IV
23. The options are to smoke or not smoke the cigarette.
24. Answers may vary. Option 1 benefit: I will impress Seth. Consequence: I will go against my values and risk my health. Option 2 benefit: I will uphold my values and avoid long-term health risks. Consequence: Seth might not want to become friends with me.
25. Answers will vary. Students may answer that smoking is undesirable because it leads to long-term health problems.
26. Answers will vary. Students may answer they would not accept the cigarette.

Chapter 2, continued

27. Answers will vary. Students might tell Seth, "No thank you, I don't smoke."

Chapter 3

Part I

1. d
2. h
3. i
4. k
5. b
6. j
7. c
8. f
9. e
10. g
11. l
12. a

Part II

13. d
14. d
15. b
16. c
17. b
18. c
19. a
20. d
21. c
22. b
23. c

Part III

24. Answers will vary. Students may answer, "I would advise my friend not to take steroids. Steroids are illegal and dangerous. They can cause high blood pressure, liver damage, cancer, damage to the reproductive system, and facial deformities. Steroids can also cause violent behavior and other psychiatric problems."

Chapter 4

Part I

1. c
2. e
3. b
4. d
5. a

Part II

6. appetite
7. health
8. hunger
9. culture
10. emotions

Part III

11. a
12. c
13. a
14. d
15. c
16. b
17. d
18. c
19. d
20. b
21. d
22. d
23. b
24. c

Part IV

25. Answers will vary. Students should point out that Lydia's diet contains too much fat, not enough carbohydrates, and limited food choices. Lydia could better meet her nutritional needs by eating more foods from the bread-cereal and vegetable-fruit groups. She should limit her intake of fatty meats and eat more lean meats, such as chicken and turkey. Lydia also needs to include foods high in iron, calcium, and vitamins B, C, and A.

Chapter 5

Part I

1. b
2. g
3. i
4. h
5. e
6. a
7. d
8. c
9. f

Part II

10. c
11. b
12. b
13. c
14. a

15. d
16. c
17. c
18. b

Part III

19. A
20. B
21. A
22. A, B
23. A
24. A, B

Part IV

25. Students should choose not to include fast foods in either diet plan. Fast foods are not usually a healthful food choice, as most are highly processed and fried, making them high in fat, calories, and sodium.

Chapter 6

Part I

1. e
2. b
3. c
4. a
5. f
6. d

Part II

7. b
8. a
9. b
10. c
11. c
12. d
13. b
14. b
15. c
16. a
17. d

Part III

18. b
19. d
20. c
21. e
22. a
23. f

Part IV

24. No. Tanning does not promote health. Exposure to ultraviolet rays can cause wrinkles, sunburn, and skin cancer. Anita will be in the sun during midday—the time when the sun's rays are the most intense. Without a sunscreen of SPF 15, she will most likely get a sunburn. People like Anita, who do not use sunscreens and who get severe sunburns, are at a higher risk for developing skin cancer.

25. Immediately wash the skin that came into contact with the plant. If you have a mild allergic reaction, obtain a cream for it from a pharmacy. If you have a severe allergic reaction, see a doctor immediately.

Chapter 7

Part I

1. h
2. d
3. c
4. a
5. g
6. j
7. i
8. e
9. f
10. b

Part II

11. d
12. c
13. b
14. c
15. d
16. d
17. a

Part III

18. phobia
19. multiple personality disorder
20. manic-depressive disorder
21. paranoid personality disorder
22. hypochondriasis
23. organic disorder
24. antisocial personality disorder

Part IV

25. No. It is normal to feel a bit anxious before a test. Since the anxiety goes away and does not interfere with a person's ability to concentrate and do well on the test, it is not causing a mental or emotional problem for the person.

Chapter 8

Part I

1. b
2. g

3. f
4. d
5. e
6. a
7. c

Part II

8. d
9. a
10. d
11. c
12. d
13. a
14. c
15. b
16. d
17. c
18. d
19. a
20. d
21. b
22. a
23. c
24. d

Part III

25. Answers will vary. Students might say that Jalene is allowing negative self-talk, and possibly media messages about how a basketball player should look, to influence her self-esteem. Students might also say that if they were Jalene and had high self-esteem, they would join in the game to have fun and make new friends and not worry so much about how they looked on the court.

Chapter 9

Part I

1. f
2. a
3. c
4. b
5. d
6. e

Part II

7. a
8. d
9. b
10. d
11. d
12. d

13. a
14. c
15. c
16. d
17. d
18. a
19. d

Part III

20. 5
21. 3
22. 1
23. 4
24. 2

Part IV

25. Answers will vary. Students may answer that they would advise Lisa to list what has to be done today and then to prioritize those things. Lisa can also say no to the baby-sitting. She might also ask another family member to help with the dishes.

Chapter 10

Part I

1. c
2. d
3. e
4. a
5. f
6. g
7. b

Part II

8. b
9. c
10. a
11. c
12. b
13. d
14. d
15. b
16. d
17. c
18. d
19. d
20. d
21. d
22. a
23. c
24. d

Part III

25. Answers will vary. Students may answer that they would assure their friend that her feelings are normal. Students may also tell their friend that it is very hard to lose someone you love and that she must miss her grandmother very much. Students may also want to assure their friend that they will be available to be with and talk with her whenever she needs them.

Chapter 11

Part I

1. c
2. d
3. a
4. b

Part II

5. d
6. b
7. d
8. c
9. a
10. d
11. a
12. c
13. d

Part III

14. M
15. M
16. F
17. F
18. M
19. M

Part IV

20. X
21.
22.
23. X
24. X

Part V

25. Answers will vary. The students might answer that Krista is showing warning signs of suicide. Maria and Steve may want to talk with Krista and ask her if she is thinking about suicide. Maria and Steve should immediately seek help for Krista by talking to a trusted adult about Krista's behavior.

Chapter 12

Part I

1. c
2. d
3. f
4. b
5. a
6. h
7. g
8. e

Part II

9. c
10. a
11. b
12. b
13. b
14. a
15. b
16. b
17. a

Part III

18. 10/15/96
19. Pamela Smith
20. Dr. Takamura
21. Home Town Pharmacy
22. One tablet 4 times daily on an empty stomach for 10 days
23. Penicillin
24. One 500 mg tablet 4 times daily
25. 10/97

Chapter 13

Part I

1. f
2. e
3. d
4. c
5. a
6. b

Part II

7. c
8. d
9. b
10. a
11. a
12. d
13. b
14. a
15. b
16. d

17. a
18. d
19. c
20. d
21. d
22. c
23. d
24. d

Part III

25. Answers will vary. Students should answer no because Becky is intoxicated. Her abilities to drive are impaired enough to cause a car crash. The students may suggest that they call their parents or get a ride home from a friend who has had no alcoholic beverages to drink.

Chapter 14

Part I

1. d
2. c
3. g
4. e
5. a
6. h
7. b
8. f

Part II

9. b
10. c
11. d
12. d
13. b
14. c
15. c
16. b
17. a
18. d
19. a
20. d
21. d
22. c
23. a

Part III

24. Answers will vary. Students might answer that one purpose of doctors and hospitals is to help ill people become well. Mainstream and sidestream smoke can cause or aggravate various diseases and disorders. Also, nonsmokers in a waiting room and those recovering in a hospital have a right to breathe clean air.

25. Answers will vary. Responses may include the following: there is a greater risk of miscarriage, the baby might be born too early, the baby might have a slow growth rate, and the baby might receive nicotine from the mother's milk.

Chapter 15

Part I

1. b
2. d
3. a
4. g
5. h
6. i
7. c
8. f
9. e

Part II

10. b
11. b
12. a
13. a
14. b
15. c
16. b
17. d
18. a
19. c
20. a
21. c
22. a
23. d
24. b

Part III

25. Answers will vary. Students may answer that they are concerned that the friend is already addicted to cocaine. They may approach the friend and talk to him about the dangers of cocaine abuse. They may also talk to him about addiction and suggest that he stop using cocaine and that he talk to someone in the Student Assistance Program at school or call a drug abuse hotline.

Chapter 16

Part I

1. b
2. i

3. e
4. i
5. f
6. g
7. h
8. d
9. a
10. c

Part II

11. b
12. d
13. c
14. a
15. d
16. b
17. a
18. d
19. d
20. d
21. b
22. d
23. b
24. d

Part III

25. 2
26. 3
27. 1
28. 5
29. 4

Part IV

30. Answers will vary. Students might respond that positive experiences, such as good relationships with parents, friendships, and accomplishments, would act to increase a person's self-esteem. Negative experiences, such as lack of parental approval, loneliness, and failures, would lower a person's self-esteem.

Chapter 17

Part I

1. c
2. g
3. f
4. h
5. e
6. d
7. b
8. a
9. j
10. i

Part II

11. d
12. d
13. c
14. b
15. a
16. b
17. b

Part III

18. facial hair
19. deeper voice
20. breasts develop
21. penis and testes increase in size
22. female organs increase in size
23. sperm production begins
24. ovulation and menstruation begin

Part IV

25. Answers will vary. Students may answer that by deciding ahead of time, you have had a chance to think of the pros and cons of sexual intimacy. You have also had a chance to work through internal and external pressures. You can practice what you might say to resist pressure before the situation arises so that you will be better prepared to stick with your decision.

Chapter 18

Part I

1. g
2. j
3. i
4. f
5. h
6. e
7. d
8. b
9. c
10. a

Part II

11. b
12. c
13. d
14. a
15. a
16. b
17. d
18. c

Part III

19. M
20. M
21. F
22. F
23. M
24. F

Part IV

25. Answers may include eating nutritious low-fat diets and exercising. This choice can lower the risk of heart disease and some cancers. Get regular physical and dental checkups and practice good hygiene. These choices can help prevent diseases and also help detect disease early so that there is a better chance for a cure. Avoid tobacco. This choice can lower the risk for cancer. Learn how to manage stress. This choice can lower the risk for heart disease and cancer as well as help maintain good mental health.

Chapter 19

Part I

1. f
2. d
3. e
4. g
5. c
6. a
7. h
8. b

Part II

9. a
10. c
11. b
12. d
13. c
14. b
15. a
16. b
17. c

Part III

18. respect for other family members
19. good communication
20. emotional support
21. share responsibility
22. manage change

Part IV

23. Students should classify the family as a healthy family that is going through a difficult time. There was no indication that the family was dysfunctional before her father lost his job. If they can manage the temporary change of her father's unemployment, they will remain a healthy family.
24. Angela would like to talk with her parents, but she doesn't feel that she can right now. Angela needs to approach her parents and discuss her concerns with them.
25. Answers may include talking to friends, a counselor, or a trusted adult.

Chapter 20

Part I

1. d
2. a
3. i
4. g
5. b
6. f
7. c
8. e
9. j
10. h

Part II

11. c
12. d
13. a
14. d
15. d
16. d
17. c
18. a
19. c
20. c
21. d
22. a

Part III

23. physical and sexual
24. Answers will vary. Students may suggest she talk with her parents, a trusted adult, or someone on the child abuse hotline. They may also suggest she report the matter to the police.
25. Answers will vary. Students may say they would report the matter to a trusted adult, such as a school nurse or counselor, or to the police.

Chapter 21

Part I

1. h
2. b
3. a
4. g
5. f
6. d
7. e
8. c

Part II

9. b
10. d
11. a
12. d
13. c
14. d
15. b
16. d
17. c
18. b
19. d

Part III

20. Virus
21. Antibiotics
22. Gamma globulin injection, rest and fluids
23. Virus
24. Virus

Part IV

25. Answers will vary. Students may answer that they can wash their hands after wiping the brother's nose with tissue, avoid putting their hands in their mouth, avoid preparing and eating foods without first washing their hands, not let the child sneeze or cough right beside them, and teach the child to cover his nose and mouth when sneezing or coughing.

Chapter 22

Part I

1. d
2. a
3. g
4. h
5. b
6. f
7. c
8. e

Part II

9. b
10. d
11. c
12. b
13. d
14. d
15. c
16. d
17. b
18. b
19. d
20. c
21. d
22. a
23. d
24. b

Part III

25. Answers will vary. Students may suggest that Angela seek testing and treatment from a doctor as soon as possible. Rob should seek testing and treatment at the same time. Rob may be infected but lack symptoms. If both of them are not treated at the same time, they will just keep reinfecting each other. STDs can only be diagnosed and treated by a doctor or a health professional at a clinic. Specific treatments are needed for specific STDs. Over-the-counter medications should not be used unless directed by a doctor. If the infection is not treated properly, it could lead to long-term consequences, such as infertility.

Chapter 23

Part I

1. e
2. b
3. h
4. a
5. f
6. g
7. d
8. c

Part II

9. b
10. c
11. b
12. d
13. c
14. b

15. a
16. a
17. c
18. b
19. b

Part III

20. R
21. S
22. R
23. S
24. S

Part IV

25. Answers will vary. Accept any response that shows an understanding of the risks involved in sexual behaviors and HIV infection and how to eliminate or reduce those risks. Sample response: Students should encourage the friend to resist pressure to have sexual intercourse and to remain abstinent. Waiting to have sexual intercourse until she is in a monogamous relationship for life is the most effective way to prevent HIV infection. They should tell the friend that condoms reduce the risk of HIV infection but do not eliminate it. Latex condoms treated with nonoxynol-9 provide the most protection against HIV. Condoms should be used with all types of sexual intercourse from start to finish.

Chapter 24

Part I

1. g
2. f
3. j
4. i
5. d
6. c
7. h
8. e
9. b
10. a

Part II

11. d
12. b
13. b
14. d
15. a
16. d
17. c

Part III

18. H
19. A
20. C
21. H
22. A
23. C
24. D

Part IV

25. A heart attack and a stroke are both cardio-vascular diseases caused by atherosclerosis or by a blood clot. When the blood supply to part of the heart is cut off, a heart attack occurs; when the blood supply to part of the brain is cut off, a stroke occurs. The damaged part of the heart and brain is replaced by scar tissue. Both a heart attack and a stroke require immediate medical treatment. A stroke can also occur when a blood vessel breaks or swells and puts pressure on the brain. The symptoms for a heart attack and a stroke differ.

Chapter 25

Part I

1. g
2. a
3. d
4. j
5. e
6. b
7. i
8. c
9. h
10. f

Part II

11. b
12. b
13. d
14. c
15. a
16. d
17. a
18. b
19. c

Part III

20. air pollution
21. water pollution
22. land pollution
23. noise pollution
24. air pollution